T0201363

The Future of Forensic Science

Published and forthcoming titles in the Forensic Science in Focus series

Published

The Global Practice of Forensic Science
Douglas H. Ubelaker (Editor)

Forensic Chemistry: Fundamentals and Applications
Jay A. Siegel (Editor)

Forensic Microbiology
David O. Carter, Jeffrey K. Tomberlin, M. Eric Benbow and
Jessica L. Metcalf (Editors)

Forensic Anthropology: Theoretical Framework and Scientific Basis
Clifford Boyd and Donna Boyd (Editors)

The Future of Forensic Science
Daniel A. Martell (Editor)

Forthcoming

Forensic Anthropology and the U. S. Judicial System
Laura C. Fulginiti, Alison Galloway and Kristen Hartnett-McCann
(Editors)

*Forensic Science and Humanitarian Action: Interacting with the Dead
and the Living*
Roberto C. Parra, Sara C. Zapico and Douglas H. Ubelaker (Editors)

Humanitarian Forensics and Human Identification
Paul Emanovsky and Shuala M. Drawdy (Editors)

The Future of Forensic Science

EDITED BY

Daniel A. Martell

Semel Institute for Neuroscience and Human Behavior
David Geffen School of Medicine at U.C.L.A.

and

Park Dietz & Associates, Inc.
Newport Beach, CA

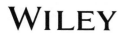

This edition first published 2019
© 2019 John Wiley & Sons Ltd

The right of Daniel A. Martell to be identified as the author of the editorial material in this work has been asserted in accordance with law.

Registered Offices
John Wiley & Sons, Inc., 111 River Street, Hoboken, NJ 07030, USA
John Wiley & Sons Ltd, The Atrium, Southern Gate, Chichester, West Sussex, PO19 8SQ, UK

Editorial Office
The Atrium, Southern Gate, Chichester, West Sussex, PO19 8SQ, UK

For details of our global editorial offices, customer services, and more information about Wiley products visit us at www.wiley.com.

Wiley also publishes its books in a variety of electronic formats and by print-on-demand. Some content that appears in standard print versions of this book may not be available in other formats.

Library of Congress Cataloging-in-Publication Data

Names: American Academy of Forensic Sciences. Interdisciplinary Symposium
   (2015 : Orlando, Fla.), author. | Martell, Daniel A. (Daniel Allen),
   editor.
Title: The future of forensic science / edited by Daniel A. Martell.
Description: First edition. | Hoboken, NJ : John Wiley & Sons, Inc., 2019. |
   Series: Forensic science in focus | Includes bibliographical references
   and index. |
Identifiers: LCCN 2018055495 (print) | LCCN 2018056614 (ebook) | ISBN
   9781119226680 (AdobePDF) | ISBN 9781119226697 (ePub) | ISBN 9781119226673
   (hardcover)
Subjects: | MESH: Forensic Sciences–trends | Congress
Classification: LCC HV8073 (ebook) | LCC HV8073 (print) | NLM W 700 | DDC
   363.25–dc23
LC record available at https://lccn.loc.gov/2018055495

Cover design: Wiley
Cover image: © Toria/Shutterstock

Set in size of 10.5/13.5pt and MeridienLTStd by SPi Global, Chennai, India
Printed in Singapore by C.O.S. Printers Pte Ltd

10 9 8 7 6 5 4 3 2 1

Contents

Notes on contributors, xi

Series preface, xix

Preface, xxi

1 New directions in forensic anthropology, 1
Douglas H. Ubelaker

1.1 Introduction, 1
1.2 Detection and recovery, 3
1.3 Determination of human status, 4
1.4 Age at death, 6
1.5 Time since death, 7
1.6 Sex estimation, 8
1.7 Ancestry, 9
1.8 Living stature, 9
1.9 Postmortem history, 10
1.10 Positive identification, 10
1.11 Foul play, 11
1.12 Certification, 12
1.13 Conclusion, 13
Acknowledgments, 14
References, 14

2 Some thoughts on the future challenges to criminalistics, 19
Ronald L. Singer

2.1 Introduction, 19
2.2 Technological advances, 20
2.2.1 Computers, software, and databases, 20
2.2.2 DNA, 21
2.2.3 Impression evidence, 21
2.2.4 Instrumentation, 22
2.3 Quality issues, 23
2.3.1 NAS Report, 23

2.4   Financial burdens, 24
    2.4.1   Seeking additional sources of grant
        funding, 25
    2.4.2   Staffing, 25
    2.4.3   Regionalization, 26
    2.4.4   Consolidation, 26
    2.4.5   Cost recovery, 27
    2.4.6   Privatization, 28
    Acknowledgments, 29
    References, 29

3 Digital and multimedia sciences, 31
Zeno Geradts

3.1   Introduction, 31
3.2   History, 33
3.3   Digital evidence, 35
3.4   Damaged (mobile) devices, 37
3.5   Multimedia, 38
    3.5.1   Deep learning (Hinton et al. 2006), 39
    3.5.2   Camera identification, 40
    3.5.3   Other biometrics, 41
3.6   Wearables and quantified self, 41
3.7   Drones, 41
3.8   Sensors, 42
3.9   Geo satellites, 42
3.10   Disasters/large scale incidents, 42
3.11   Quality assurance, 43
3.12   Challenges, 43
    References, 44

4 A look at the future of forensic engineering science, 49
Thomas L. Bohan

    "The future": a preface, 49
4.1   Junk law in the courtroom, 50
4.2   Forensic engineering sciences and needs of the
    modern world at large, 55
    Acknowledgments, 58
    References, 58

5 General section history: look at two disciplines and a review of standards, certifications, and education, 61
John E. Gerns

5.1 Introduction, 61
5.2 Forensic veterinary science, 62
5.3 Certification: introduction, 66
5.4 Certification—ABMDI, 66
5.5 Standards evolution—OSAC, 68
5.6 Standard evolution—ASB, 69
5.7 Education accreditation, 70
5.8 Summary, 71
 Acknowledgements, 72
 References, 72

6 The future of forensic science: hot leads in contemporary forensic research: Jurisprudence, 73
Carol Henderson

6.1 Daubert's history, 75
6.2 The *Daubert* test, 77
6.3 Questions raised by *Daubert*, 77
6.4 The NAS report, 78
6.5 The national commission on forensic science and the organization of scientific area committees, 80
6.6 NCFS, 80
6.7 OSAC, 82
6.8 The path forward for judicial and legal education in forensic science, 84
 Acknowledgments, 87
 References, 87

7 Forensic odontology, 91
Robert E. Barsley

7.1 Introduction, 91
7.2 Roles of the forensic odontologist, 92
7.3 Current considerations, 94
7.4 Identification by teeth, 96
7.5 Dental age assessment, 104
7.6 Bitemarks, 105

7.7   Abuse and negligence, 107

7.8   Closing, 107

8 Opportunities and problems faced in forensic pathology, 109
Edmund R. Donoghue

8.1   Opportunity: radiology technology and computer imaging, 109

8.2   Threat: dropping forensic pathology training requirement for anatomic pathology, 110

8.3   Threat: maintenance of certification could see some forensic pathologists unemployed, 111

8.4   Threat: standards are becoming increasingly detailed and rigorous, 112

8.5   Threat: forensic: overregulation by federal government and other entities, 112

8.6   Conclusion, 112

9 The future of forensic psychiatry and behavioral science, 113
Richard Rosner

9.1   The BRAIN initiative, 114

9.2   The law and the human mind, 114

9.3   Correlation is NOT causation, 115

9.4   Theories of consciousness, 115

9.5   The hard problem of consciousness, 116

9.6   Consciousness and the failure of the physical sciences, 117

9.7   The problem of free will, 118

9.8   The bottom line, 119
      References, 119

10 The future of forensic document examination, 121
John L. Sang, Linton A. Mohammed and Carl R. McClary

10.1   What is a forensic document examiner (FDE)?, 121

10.2   Origins of questioned document examination, 123

10.3   Albert S. Osborn and the formation of the American Society of Questioned Document Examiners (ASQDE), 125

10.4   Ordway Hilton and the formation of American
       Academy of Forensic Sciences (AAFS), 126
10.5   Questioned documents and the formation of the
       International Association of Forensic Sciences
       (IAFS), 128
10.6   Key issues, 128
       10.6.1   Certification, 128
       10.6.2   Standardization, 129
10.7   Standards of practice, 132
10.8   The Daubert standard and FDE, 135
10.9   How FDE meets Daubert, 137
       10.9.1   Standards, 137
       10.9.2   Error rate/reliability, 138
       10.9.3   Testing of basic principles, 139
       10.9.4   Peer review and publication, 142
       10.9.5   General acceptance in the forensic
                community, 143
10.10 Research in FDE, 144
       10.10.1 Neuroscience, 144
       10.10.2 Eye tracking, 146
10.11 Signature and handwriting verification
       systems, 148
10.12 Automation in the forensic examination of
       handwriting, 148
10.13 Current research, 149
10.14 Conclusion, 150
       10.14.1 The public and how law and forensics will
                be shaped, 150
       10.14.2 Research, 151
       10.14.3 Research in other document
                examinations, 151
       References, 152
       Further readings, 155
       Measurement science and standards in forensic
       handwriting analysis – U.S. Commerce Department's
       National Institute of Standards and Technology
       (NIST) Symposium, June 2013 presentations, 157

11 Past perspectives and future directions in forensic toxicology, 159
Barry K. Logan F-ABFT

11.1   Our history, 159
11.2   Reflections on factors affecting our future
        direction, 163
11.3   Facing forward, 167
        11.3.1   Laboratory resources and the role of the
                  Federal Government, 168
        11.3.2   Standards development and harmonization
                  of best practices, 168
        11.3.3   Technology, 169
        11.3.4   Training, research, and interdisciplinary
                  collaboration, 171
11.4   Conclusion, 173
        Acknowledgments, 174

Index, 175

Notes on contributors

Bob Barsley, has been continually licensed in Louisiana to practice dentistry since 1977 and to practice law since 1987. He is a tenured Professor at LSU where he has been full-time faculty since 1882. He is a fellow of the American College of Dentists, the International College of Dentists, the Pierre Fauchard Academy, and the Odontology Section of the American Academy of Forensic Sciences. He has also served as a Robert Wood Johnson Foundation Congressional Health Policy Fellow in the office of Senator John Breaux. He is a past president, past Speaker of the House, and a past secretary/treasurer of the Louisiana Dental Association. He is the immediate past Chair of the Council of Scientific Society Presidents in Washington, DC.

Dr. Barsley has also served as Acting State Dental Director of the Louisiana Office of Public Health and as the Chief Compliance Office for the LSU Health Sciences Center. He has held numerous officers in various forensic organizations and is a past president of the American Academy of Forensic Sciences, past Treasurer of the Forensic Science Foundation, and is a past president of the American Board of Forensic Odontology and of the American Society of Forensic Odontology. He has been a member of the *Journal of Forensic Sciences* Editorial Board for many years and is a frequent guest reviewer for the *Journal of the American Dental Association* and the *Journal of Dental Education*. He was named by NIST to chair the Odontology Subcommittee of the Organization of Scientific Area Committees under the auspices of the Forensic Sciences Standards Board. He served as the magistrate judge for the Ponchatoula City Court for nine years.

Thomas L. Bohan, Ph.D., J.D., holds his physics PhD from the University of Illinois-Urbana/Champaign and his law degree from the University of New Hampshire School of Law. He has authored books and peer-reviewed papers in the scientific and legal professional literature. Reflecting his interest in forensic science and its admission into evidence, these publications include early commentary on the Daubert decision and an extensive review of the 2009 National Academy of Science report Forensic Science in the United States.

While president of the American Academy of Forensic Sciences (2009–2010), he sought to make the Academy a partner in the forensic-science reform called from by the report. Later, while president of the Forensic Specialties Accreditation Board (2015–2017), he oversaw the revision of that organization's standards so as to limit the board's offer of accreditation to those Conformity Assessment Bodies that certified forensic practices that are reliable and reproducible. He resides in Casco Bay's Peaks Island in the State of Maine.

Edmund R. Donoghue, M.D. is a forensic pathologist and regional medical examiner for the Georgia Bureau of Investigation in Savannah, GA. Dr. Donoghue is a graduate of the University of Notre Dame and the Medical College of Wisconsin. He received postgraduate medical specialty training at the Mayo Clinic, the Wayne County Medical Examiner's Office, and the Armed Forces Institute of Pathology. For 30 years he was employed by the Office of the Medical Examiner of Cook County in Chicago, IL, and for the last 14 of those years he was chief medical examiner.

Dr. Donoghue is certified by the American Board of Pathology in anatomic and forensic pathology. He served as a clinical professor of forensic pathology at the University of Illinois at Chicago. He has served as president and chair of the board of directors of the National Association of Medical Examiners. Dr. Donoghue is a past president of the Chicago Medical Society, the Georgia Medical Society, and the American Academy of Forensic Sciences.

Zeno Geradts is a senior forensic scientist at the department of Digital and Biometric Traces of the Netherlands Forensic Institute. He is for one day a week full professor by special chair of forensic data science at the University of Amsterdam. His research interests are the use of deep learning and artificial intelligence in forensic science in interpreting images and data.

He is president elect of the American Academy of Forensic Sciences 2018–2019 and will be the 2019–2020 president of the AAFS. Furthermore, he is associate editor of the *Journal of Forensic Sciences,* and chairman of the European Network of Forensic Science (ENFSI) Forensic IT working group.

John Gerns is past president of the AAFS and sat on the AAFS Executive Committee and the board of directors. He has been with the AAFS since 1983 and became a Fellow in 1992. He is an Adjunct Professor for Central Texas College and the University of Maryland University College where he teaches Forensic Science and Criminal Justice. In addition, he provides forensic science consultation on violent crimes.

Prior to his retirement on 30 September 2013, he was the Investigations and Operations Consultant assigned to the Fourth Field Investigations Squadron, Vogelweh, Germany. He has extensive training and experience in major investigations involving death, child physical and sexual abuse, sexual assault, mass grave exhumations, along with crime scene processing and reconstruction. Special Agent Gerns' assignments have included Command Forensic Advisor, Director of Criminal Investigations, Director of Investigative Specialties, Forensic Consultant to International Criminal Tribunal for the former Yugoslavia (ICTY), and Chief of Death Investigations. His primary role during that period was ensuring the latest innovations in the forensic sciences were applied to AFOSI's investigative mission.

Carol Henderson is the founding director of the National Clearinghouse for Science, Technology, and the Law, and a professor of law at Stetson University College of Law. Professor Henderson has presented more than 300 lectures and workshops worldwide on scientific evidence, courtroom testimony, and professional responsibility. She has more than 90 publications including "Sleuthing Scientific Evidence Information on the Internet," 106 *Journal of Criminal Law and Criminology*59 (2016) and "Future Focus for Forensic Science," a special issue of *The Sci Tech Lawyer* (2017).

Professor Henderson has appeared in national media as a legal analyst and testified before the US Congress. She served as the president of the American Academy of Forensic Sciences (2008–2009) and presently serves on the ABA's Science and Technology Law Section Council. She is the deputy editor-in-chief of *The SciTech Lawyer*. She also serves on the ABA Judicial Division Forensic Science Committee and as faculty for the National Judicial College. In February 2019, she received the American Academy of Forensic Sciences Distinguished Fellow award.

Barry K. Logan PhD, is chief scientist at NMS Labs and executive director of the Center for Forensic Science Research and Education in Willow Grove PA. He has authored or coauthored over 120 publications, and his current research interests are in the area of Novel Psychoactive Substances, and Drug and Alcohol Impaired Driving.

He holds academic appointments at Indiana University, where he directs the Robert F. Borkenstein Course on Alcohol, and at Thomas Jefferson University where he is director of the Forensic Toxicology Professional Science Masters Program. He served as president of the American Academy of Forensic Sciences between 2013 and 2014.

Daniel A. Martell, Ph.D., A.B.P.P. is a forensic neuropsychologist who has specialized experience applying diverse knowledge to cases involving forensic neuroscience and human behavior. He is Board-Certified in Forensic Psychology by the American Board of Professional Psychology; a Fellow of the American Academy of Forensic Psychology; and a Fellow of the National Academy of Neuropsychology; a Fellow of the Royal Society of Medicine in London; and a Fellow and Past President of the American Academy of Forensic Sciences.

He is a member of the Clinical Faculty in the Department of Psychiatry and Biobehavioral Sciences at the Semel Institute for Neuroscience and Human Behavior at the David Geffen School of Medicine at UCLA.

Examples of his expertise in criminal cases include brain damage and crimes of violence, mass murderers and serial killers, violent sexual predators, and capital habeas corpus appeals litigation. He is particularly experienced with dozens of cases involving determinations of Intellectual Disability and the death penalty pursuant to *Atkins v. Virginia*, having been the prosecution's expert in that landmark case. His experience in civil litigation includes damages determinations in mass torts, lawsuits arising from clergy abuse, corporate civil and products liability, employment law, and elder law cases involving testamentary capacity and undue influence.

Carl R. McClary is a senior forensic document examiner and technical lead with the Bureau of Alcohol, Tobacco, Firearms, and Explosives forensic science laboratory in Atlanta, Georgia. He is a member of the Questioned Documents consensus body of the Academy Standards Board (ASB) and former chair of the E30.02 Questioned Documents subcommittee of the American Society for Testing and Materials International (ASTM). Some of his recent research focus has been on document examiner aptitude in determining stroke velocity rates in handwriting, opinion terminology standardization, and forensic science training development and standardization. He is the current treasurer of the American Academy of Forensic Sciences.

Linton A. Mohammed, Ph.D., D-ABFDE has been in the field of Forensic Document Examination for more than 30 years. His PhD thesis was entitled "Elucidating spatial and dynamic features to discriminate between signature disguise and signature forgery behavior." He has testified as an expert witness more than 100 times in the United States, England, and the Caribbean. He is the coauthor of "The Neuroscience of Handwriting: Applications for Forensic Document Examination," and has published several papers in peer-reviewed journals. Dr. Mohammed has conducted or copresented workshops on signature and document examination in Australia, Brazil, Canada, China, Latvia, Poland, Saudi Arabia, Turkey, and the United States. In 2012, he was given the New Horizon Award in Recognition of Exceptional Contributions in Scientific Research for the Advancement of Forensic Document Examination by the American Board of Forensic Document Examiners, Inc.

Dr. Mohammed is certified by the American Board of Forensic Document Examiners, Inc. and holds a Diploma in Document Examination from the Chartered Society of Forensic Sciences. He is a member and past president of the American Society of Questioned Document Examiners, Inc., a Fellow of the Questioned Documents Section of the American Academy of Forensic Sciences and serving as the Chair of the Section from 2016 to 2018. He serves on the Editorial Review Boards of the *Journal of Forensic Sciences* and *Journal of the American Society of Questioned Document Examiners*, and is a guest reviewer for several other journals. Dr. Mohammed is in private practice in Burlingame, CA (San Francisco Bay Area).

Richard Rosner, M.D. is a clinical professor of Psychiatry and a clinical professor of Child and Adolescent Psychiatry at New York University School of Medicine. He is editor or coeditor of nine books on forensic psychiatry and three books on adolescent psychiatry. He is a former president and distinguished fellow of the American Academy of Forensic Sciences (AAFS). The AAFS Psychiatry and Behavioral Science Section named its annual award for the Best Paper by a Forensic Psychiatry Fellow or a Forensic Psychology Fellow in his honor, that is, the Richard Rosner Award.

He is a former president of the American Academy of Psychiatry and the Law (AAPL). He has received AAPL's Seymour Pollack award for teaching, AAPL's "Red Apple" award for services to the organization, and AAPL's "Golden Apple" for lifetime achievements in forensic psychiatry. He has been president of the Accreditation Council on Fellowships in Forensic Psychiatry and president of the Association of Directors of Forensic Psychiatry Fellowships. He is a former president of the American Board of Forensic Psychiatry, Inc. He is a distinguished life fellow of the American Psychiatric Association (APA). He is a recipient of the Isaac Ray Award of the APA for distinguished contributions to forensic psychiatry. He (with Charles Scott, M.D.) received the Manfred Guttmacher Award of the APA for their book *Principles and Practice of Forensic Psychiatry*, Third Edition. He is a fellow of the American College of Psychiatrists. He is a fellow of the American Society for Adolescent Psychiatry (ASAP), a former president of ASAP, a recipient of the Herman Staples Award for distinguished services to ASAP, and a recipient of the highest recognition bestowed by ASAP, its William Schoenfeld Award.

Douglas H. Ubelaker, Ph.D. is a curator and senior scientist at the Smithsonian Institution's National Museum of Natural History in Washington, DC. where he has been employed for over four decades. Since 1978, he has served as a consultant in forensic anthropology. In this capacity, he has served as an expert witness, reporting on more than 980 cases and has testified in numerous legal proceedings.

He is a professorial lecturer with the Departments of Anatomy and Anthropology at the George Washington University, Washington, DC., and is an adjunct professor with the Department of Anthropology,

Michigan State University, East Lansing, Michigan. Dr. Ubelaker has published extensively in the general field of human skeletal biology with an emphasis on forensic applications. He served as the 2011–2012 president of the AAFS.

John Sang received his Master of Science from the Forensic Science Program at John Jay College of Criminal Justice, The City University of New York. He served as vice president of the American Academy of Forensic Sciences 2010–2011 and four years on the board of directors and served as Section Chair of the Question Documents Section. He chaired many technical workshops at the AAFS. He received the American Academy of Forensic Sciences Question Document Sections Ordway Hilton Award in Recognition of Outstanding Contributions to Forensic Document Examination. He was certified by American Board of Forensic Document Examination (ABFDE), is a Member of the American Society of Testing and Materials International and the Northeastern Association of Forensic Sciences.

John taught at John Jay College of Criminal Justice, University of New Haven, Ct., Brooklyn Law School, Brooklyn, NY, New York City Police Academy, Advanced and Specialized Training and the NYPD Crime Laboratory. He was a lieutenant with the New York City Police Department with specialties in scientific and criminal investigation. He served as technical supervisor and as a forensic document examiner in the Forensic Document Section of the New York City Police Crime Laboratory. He had a number of other positions in the Police Department and testified in a number of high-profile cases. He is now in private practice as a Forensic Document Examiner.

Ronald L. Singer, M.S. is the technical and administrative director for the Tarrant County (Texas) Medical Examiner's Office. A forensic scientist for over 46 years, he is a distinguished fellow and past president of the American Academy of Forensic Sciences; a distinguished member and past president of the Association of Firearm and Tool Mark Examiners, and a past president of the International Association of Forensic Science.

He is the recipient of the American Academy of Forensic Sciences Criminalistics Section Distinguished Service Award, the Mediterranean Academy of Forensic Sciences Gold Medal Award and the

Association of Firearm and Tool Mark Examiners Member of the Year Award, and has been an invited speaker throughout the United States and England, Hungary, Bosnia, the Maldives, Sri Lanka, Turkey, the Czech Republic, Portugal, Dubai, and Lebanon.

Series preface

The forensic sciences represent diverse, dynamic fields that seek to utilize the very best techniques available to address legal issues. Fueled by advances in technology, research, and methodology, as well as new case applications, the forensic sciences continue to evolve. Forensic scientists strive to improve their analyses and interpretations of evidence and to remain cognizant of the latest advancements. This series results from a collaborative effort between the American Academy of Forensic Sciences (AAFS) and Wiley to publish a select number of books that relate closely to the activities and Objectives of the AAFS. The book series reflects the goals of the AAFS to encourage quality scholarship and publication in the forensic sciences. Proposals for publication in the series are reviewed by a committee established for that purpose by the AAFS and also reviewed by Wiley.

The AAFS was founded in 1948 and represents a multidisciplinary professional organization that provides leadership to advance science and its application to the legal system. The 11 sections of the AAFS consist of Criminalistics, Digital and Multimedia Sciences, Engineering Sciences, General, Pathology/Biology, Questioned Documents, Jurisprudence, Anthropology, Toxicology, Odontology, and Psychiatry and Behavioral Science. There are over 7000 members of the AAFS, originating from all 50 states of the United States and many countries beyond. This series reflects global AAFS membership interest in new research, scholarship, and publication in the forensic sciences.

Douglas H. Ubelaker
Smithsonian Institution
Washington, DC, USA
November, 2018

Preface

This book captures the content of the 2015 American Academy of Forensic Sciences (AAFS) Interdisciplinary Symposium, one of the highlights of the Academy meeting in Orlando, FL. Preeminent visionaries in their respective fields, this collection of authors are all past presidents and officers of the AAFS, and as such provide a diverse interdisciplinary view of the direction forensics will take in the years to come. These experts are not only familiar with the past in their fields but are also looking forward to the future to envision where forensic science will be a decade from now.

The past presidents of the AAFS represent a vast repository of forensic science experience, knowledge, insight, and wisdom. As a group, they are unique in the world with regard to the scope of their collective influence and leadership vision in the forensic sciences. This volume, based on the 2015 AAFS Interdisciplinary Symposium, harnesses the energy from this eminent group of forensic scientists and focuses it on the Academy's future.

Here, the authors share their vision for the future of forensic science in their respective disciplines, emphasizing hot leads from the laboratory, theoretical advances, and emerging technologies. The goal of this volume is to envision where the forensic sciences will be a decade from now, the impact of these emerging advances on the law, and our place in it. This historic endeavor will be of significant interest to all Academy members and provides a unique forum for learning from each other about the future of forensic science.

At a time when there is enormous international interest in the future of forensic science, from articulating standards to the evolution of scientific methods, instrumentation, and technologies, the need for leadership is critical. This book provides an opportunity to provide that leadership to the entire forensic science community. The authors represented in this volume comprise some of the greatest forensic minds of their generation; leaders who command the respect and admiration of the entire international forensic community. The opportunity to gather them together and focus their energies on a vision for the future of our field is both invaluable and unprecedented.

There has never been a volume that brings together such a broad spectrum of renowned thought leaders in all areas of forensic science. The high profile of the authors, the fact that all 11 sections of the AAFS are represented, the broad appeal of the topic to an international audience, and the timing that coincides with the NIST forensic science initiative and the OSAC process all contribute to the importance and appeal of this volume.

It has been my great honor to join this group and help to shape and coordinate this endeavor.

Daniel A. Martell
American Academy of Forensic Sciences

CHAPTER 1

New directions in forensic anthropology

Douglas H. Ubelaker

Smithsonian Institution, Department of Anthropology, National Museum of Natural History, Washington, DC, USA

1.1 Introduction

Forensic anthropology represents the application of knowledge and methodology within anthropology to medicolegal issues. This process usually involves the detection, recovery, and analysis of materials that were thought to represent human skeletal remains. Analysis focuses on determining if the materials are in fact human remains, and if so, gleaning information about the individual they represent. Central goals in this effort are aimed at personal positive identification and detection of foul play.

Academic roots of the field extend back into nineteenth century European centers of anatomy and medicine. Advances in comparative anatomy, anthropometry, and growth and development by such pioneers as Paul Broca (1824–1880), Alphonse Bertillon (1853–1914), and Johann Friedrich Blumenbach (1752–1840) laid the European foundation for later advances. In the United States, two high-profile trials, the Parkman murder trial relating to a death at Harvard University in Massachusetts and the Chicago-based Adolph Luetgert trial brought widespread attention to the nascent field of forensic anthropology. These legal events involved testimony by Harvard professors Oliver Wendell Homes (1809–1894) and Jefferies Wyman (1814–1874) and the Chicago-based anthropologist George A. Dorsey (1868–1931). Research specifically targeting problems in forensic anthropology was initiated by the pioneers Thomas Dwight

The Future of Forensic Science, First Edition. Edited by Daniel A. Martell.
© 2019 John Wiley & Sons Ltd. Published 2019 by John Wiley & Sons Ltd.

(1843–1911), H.H. Wilder (1864–1928), Paul Stevenson (1890–1971), Earnest A. Hooton (1887–1954), T. Wingate Todd (1885–1938), and Smithsonian anthropologist Aleš Hrdlička (1869–1943) among others. The modern era with a specific focus on forensic anthropology as an academic area of anthropology and forensic science was ushered in by Wilton M. Krogman (1903–1987) and T. D. Stewart (1901–1997) with key contributions also by Mildred Trotter (1899–1991). Organizational advances included the 1972 effort to form a new section of the American Academy of Forensic Sciences and the 1977/1978 establishment of the American Board of Forensic Anthropology, largely through the leadership of past AAFS President Ellis R. Kerley (1924–1998). Clyde C. Snow (1928–2014) became involved in identification efforts in Latin America in 1984 and advanced global anthropological involvement in humanitarian and human rights investigations relating to anthropology. These pioneers and early initiatives coupled with abundant published research and casework established the foundation of the current field of forensic anthropology.

Although contemporary forensic anthropology is generally regarded as a subdiscipline within the more general areas of forensic science and anthropology, it really involves a conglomerate of applications and methodologies that are problem-specific. These areas of application include detection, recovery, determination of human status, estimation of age at death, time since death, sex, ancestry and living stature, assessment of postmortem history, positive identification, and evaluation of evidence for foul play. Each of the major areas of application within forensic anthropology presents its own methodology, individual historical development, and research issues (Steadman 2013). Collectively, they also require broad training and experience that is usually captured in various ways in the skills of individual practitioners.

This chapter examines methodological issues within each of the areas of application. Current techniques and developments are noted. However, since the nature of forensic anthropology and its applications are rapidly evolving, emerging issues and likely future solutions are emphasized (Lesciotto 2015).

1.2 Detection and recovery

Many cases within the field of forensic anthropology begin with efforts to detect the presence of human remains. Roots of these efforts usually stem from investigative information regarding past events suggesting the possible or likely presence of human remains. Although the nature of such cases is highly variable, a classic scenario would involve an informant indicating he witnessed a past homicide and providing general details regarding the location of burial of the decedent. The anthropologist might serve as a team consultant/participant to assist in organizing the search and advising on what methodological approaches might be utilized. If a specific location is found or targeted, the anthropologist should organize or conduct the excavation or particular detection effort. In such scenarios, it is important that the anthropologist participate in the detection effort to immediately recognize the presence of human remains if encountered.

As with most areas of application in forensic anthropology, the selection of search and detection methods depends on the issues presented by the particular case (Cheetham and Hanson 2009). The size of the search area, quality of the investigative information, topography and nature of the terrain, and availability of supportive equipment and personnel represent key variables. Possible approaches include pedestrian survey, aerial survey, and the use of cadaver dogs (Holland and Connell 2009). Land surface searches usually seek physical evidence (human remains, clothing, other artifacts, etc.) or evidence of past soil disturbance that might indicate human burial. Past soil disturbance may present detectable variation in the normal topography. Significant variants may include depressions, mounds, or unusual vegetation patterns.

In recent years, traditional survey techniques have been supplemented with technological advancement. Examples include ground-penetrating radar, soil resistivity, and magnetometry. Each of these applications seeks variations in soil patterns that might represent the soil disturbance associated with human burial. They are ideally utilized in homogeneous environments with minimal soil disturbance.

Once a specific site of possible human burial has been located, detailed excavation is called for. The forensic anthropologist trained in archeological techniques is uniquely qualified to conduct this work. The goal is to define the limits of the original burial and locate, document, and recover all relevant evidence, especially human remains and associated artifacts. Proper excavation is needed to minimize damage to the evidence and to document patterns and associations. Such work, conducted properly, maximizes the potential of later interpretation.

The nature of search and recovery efforts varies tremendously with the issues presented by each case. Although the approaches discussed previously are generally relevant, specific applications must target the individuality of the case. Scenes can vary from the classic human burial described previously to underwater environments, the aftermath of building fires, natural disasters, political conflicts, airplane crashes, and others.

Although technological advances in this area of forensic anthropology have been both impressive and useful, in my view, the primary advancement has been (and will continue to be) the growing inclusion of anthropologists in search and recovery efforts. Leadership in search and recovery teams increasingly understands the value of including the skilled anthropologist when human remains may be anticipated.

1.3 Determination of human status

A primary step in forensic anthropological analysis of recovered materials consists of determining if human remains are present. If intact bones or teeth are detected, then this task is easily accomplished through morphological examination (Mulhern 2009). However, in many cases, evidence is fragmentary and/or has been compromised by thermal events, trauma, antemortem disease, or other factors making morphological assessment difficult. In many forensic evidence situations such as recovered fire debris, it can be difficult to distinguish fragments of bone and tooth from other materials. Recent technological advances have greatly augmented anthropological capability to accurately evaluate such evidence.

Techniques of scanning electron microscopy/energy dispersive spectroscopy (SEM/EDS) are especially useful to separate fragments of bone and tooth from other similarly appearing materials. Bones and teeth contain proportions of calcium and phosphorus that differ from other materials commonly recovered in scenes (Zimmerman et al. 2015). Comparative databases have been established for the composition of these materials enabling a definitive diagnosis for the presence of bone or tooth following SEM/EDS analysis (Ubelaker et al. 2002). However, since humans and other animals share chemical composition of their bones and teeth, this approach will not lead to species determination.

To determine species represented by bone or tooth, a variety of approaches are available. Histological examination may reveal features (plexiform bone or osteon-banding patterns) that are not present in humans. However, the human histological pattern is shared with many nonhuman animals usually precluding definitive diagnosis of human status.

Molecular analysis of bone or tooth samples may reveal the species represented. This approach utilizing mitochondrial DNA markers has been employed successfully in wildlife forensic science, especially related to game and commercial species of legal interest (Guglich et al. 1994).

In my view, an ideal technique in such cases consists of solid-phase double-antibody protein radioimmunoassay (pRIA). This technique involves the extraction of protein from very small samples of the unknown specimen. The protein is then exposed in a two-phase process to species-specific antibodies. The extent of the species-specific antibody reaction can be measured through an associated radioactive marker. The technique can not only determine if human remains are present but also the likely nonhuman species present. The amount of sample required for the analysis is so small, that enough remains for molecular analysis if the pRIA analysis determines that human species is present (Ubelaker et al. 2004).

Future progress in this area of forensic anthropology likely will involve making this technology more economical and mobile. Great advancement would be made if those working in scene recovery could immediately determine the species status of recovered fragments.

1.4   Age at death

In the analysis of human skeletal remains, forensic anthropologists attempt to create a biological profile of the individual represented in order to facilitate the search for identification (Rogers 2009). Accurate estimation of the age at death is an essential component of this process. Age at death usually represents a known feature of missing persons and is thus an important element of any attempt at identification. Methodology utilized to estimate age at death varies depending upon the aspects of the remains present and the general age of the individual. For fetal remains, long bone lengths can be used to estimate body length and age using published regression equations. For infants, children, and adolescents, bone size and maturation provide some information, but the most reliable estimates are derived from evaluations of dental formation.

In recent years, the process of evaluating age at death has progressed through the acquisition of new methods, critical evaluation of existing methods, and greater awareness of the impact of population variation (Merritt 2014; Wink 2014; De Angelis et al. 2015). New methodology continues to explore not only areas of the skeleton exhibiting age-related change, but also existing techniques in other areas of science show promise in forensic application (Mays 2014; Boyd et al. 2015). An example of the latter consists of quantification of mtDNA mutations. Such mutations have been documented as playing an important role in human aging but only recently have been considered for their forensic applications (Zapico and Ubelaker 2013a).

Critical evaluation of methodology represents an essential ingredient in quality forensic science. In anthropology, it is especially important to test established methods in regard to new applications and in consideration of likely population variation (Moraitis et al. 2014; Shirley and Ramirez Montes 2015). Assessment of the impact of population variation in age at death estimation is facilitated by the increasing availability of documented skeletal collections in different global regions (Ubelaker 2014a). Many such studies document that population variation does exist in the process of human aging. This research suggests that population-specific standards should be employed when available.

Future research in age at death estimation likely will focus on the issues discussed previously. Goals include acquisition of data and samples more adequately reflecting global population variation. Such data probably will emerge from studies of newly assembled documented skeletal collections as well as increasing research on the living. Investigators will also concentrate on more robust quantification of the probabilities involved in age estimation (Villa et al. 2015). Accurate statistical presentations are needed to more realistically convey the associated variation and to satisfy increasing scrutiny in the legal arena.

1.5   Time since death

When human remains are found, authorities need to know as accurately as possible the date of death. Unfortunately, when remains are skeletonized, research and casework have demonstrated the difficulty of accurate estimation from morphology due to the myriad of variables involved. Climate, seasonality, soil conditions, individual constitution, mortuary treatment, ground water levels, extent and type of clothing and containers, accessibility to insects and scavengers, and many other factors can dramatically affect the extent of tissue preservation (Forbes and Nugent 2009; Kanz et al. 2014). In short, when remains are skeletonized and information is lacking of these variables, it is not possible to produce an accurate estimate from observations of tissue preservation. Considerable perspective has been acquired through experimentation and observations at various decay facilities, especially in consideration of local environmental issues and degree days of exposure (Dabbs 2015; Roberts and Dabbs 2015). Nevertheless, if remains are skeletonized or display environmentally induced unusual soft tissue preservation, morphology alone does not permit accurate estimates of time since death.

Radiocarbon analysis represents an attractive solution to this problem. Carbon-14 dating has long been utilized in archeological applications to securely date recovered samples. This application is based on the knowledge that the carbon-14 isotope is mildly radioactive with a known half-life of 5730 years. In the traditional application, the extent of decay is quantified and used to calculate the antiquity prior to the modern value of 1950 CE. If decay is detected, traditional analysis will reveal the great antiquity of the remains and usually exclude them from the need for medicolegal analysis.

If the remains are modern, both the birth date and death date potentially can be established through comparison of the modern radiocarbon values with the documented post-1950 bomb-curve of atmospheric levels. After 1950, the amount of base radiocarbon in the atmosphere and food chain increased dramatically until about 1965 due to atmospheric testing of thermal nuclear devices. While the levels have decreased since 1965, they continue to remain above those present prior to 1950. Thus, if the elevated levels are found, they indicate the organism was alive after 1950. Birth date and death date may be estimated from a comparison of the elevated levels with the bomb-curve, in consideration of the tissues sampled and the estimated age at death of the individual (Ubelaker et al. 2006; Ubelaker 2014b).

Future research likely will concentrate on the variables involved in radiocarbon analysis, especially the lag time (difference between atmospheric levels and those in human tissues) association with age of the individual and the variation presented in different skeletal and dental tissues. Attention also is needed on how other isotope markers of the period of modern bomb testing can be utilized to assess the death date.

1.6   Sex estimation

Since sex is almost always known in regard to characteristics of missing persons, it, like age at death, represents an important component of the biological profile. If the pelvis is available, in most cases, sex can be reliably estimated from adult skeletal morphology. Sex estimation is less reliable if the pelvis is absent or damaged since sexual dimorphism in other bones is size-related and presents some variation (Fateh et al. 2014; Michel et al. 2015). In general, sex estimation from bone morphology is not reliable in immature remains. Molecular analysis, particularly amelogenin testing, offers a reliable alternative to morphological assessment, even with immature remains (Baker 2009).

Considerable research has been conducted on sexual variation in the morphology of many individual bones of the skeleton (Wescott 2015). Such information is important since in many cases, skeletons are incomplete and may even consist of individual bones (Ostrofsky and Churchill 2015).

Research also has established considerable population variation in the expression of sexual dimorphism in the human skeleton (Brzobohatá et al. 2015). Studies originating from global samples of documented human remains gradually have made available population-specific data on sex differences (Spradley et al. 2015). As with other applications in forensic anthropology, sex estimation from bone morphology should employ local standards (Amores et al. 2014).

Future work is needed to further clarify population variation regarding sex differences in various aspects of the human skeleton. Research is also needed for additional clarification of the probabilities involved. Investigations also may discover sex differences in other tissues and substances within preserved human remains that might prove useful (Zapico and Ubelaker 2013b).

1.7 Ancestry

Evaluation of ancestry represents one of the most challenging applications of forensic anthropology (Hefner and Ousley 2014). Methodology involves both metric and nonmetric approaches and has advanced with the formation of new databases and useful customized regression formulae (Sauer and Wankmiller 2009; Pilloud et al. 2014; Klales and Kenyhercz 2015).

An important advancement has been the recognition that community ancestry classifications relate social/historical issues, as well as biological factors. Future progress likely will involve enhanced regional databases but will continue to respect the social dimensions involved.

1.8 Living stature

Current methods to estimate living stature in adults involve applications of sex and ancestry-specific regression equations to individual bones or groups of bones and also, in cases involving complete skeletons, measuring those bones that contribute to living stature (Willey 2009). Research has demonstrated the greater accuracy of the latter approach, but it is limited by frequently encountered incomplete remains. Since body proportions are known to vary considerably between the sexes and in different populations, formulae are sex and population-specific. Increasing global availability of skeletons from individuals of documented living stature has facilitated the formulation of new population-specific formulae. Also, important has been the increased recognition of the likely errors involved in the estimated statures of missing persons.

Progress in stature estimations likely will occur in (i) the availability of new formulae for different bones from more populations and (ii) more nuanced use of "known" statures from missing persons.

1.9 Postmortem history

In the forensic context, taphonomy represents the study of factors contributing to postmortem alterations of human remains (Nawrocki 2009). This area of forensic investigation recognizes that postmortem change can be influenced by many different factors. Although these influences complicate the estimation of time since death, details may reveal useful indicators of postmortem events. Animal gnaw marks, evidence of sun exposure, vegetation residue, adhering soil particles, associated arthropod remains as well as tool marks all may provide critical evidence needed to interpret the postmortem history of human remains (Young et al. 2015).

The field of taphonomy has attracted considerable research attention, leading to a growing scientific literature. Research includes a variety of innovative experiments providing a greater understanding of the impact of environmental agents on the postmortem condition of human remains.

1.10 Positive identification

Much of the forensic investigation summarized is directed toward the goal of positive individual identification. Usually, this process involves comparing the discovered individual attributes of recovered human remains with those of missing persons. Once the search is narrowed, possibly relating the remains to a few missing persons with the necessary shared characteristics, detailed analysis is conducted to ascertain if an identification can be made. Positive identification requires that unique features are found to be shared between the recovered remains and a particular missing person. In the practice of forensic anthropology, this evidence usually originates from radiographs or related medical images of bone structure.

Proper identification is a two-step procedure. First, features must be found that are shared between the recovered remains and a missing person. The second step must explain any differences that occur and assess the uniqueness of the shared attributes. Positive identification results when differences can be successfully reconciled and the shared features are judged to be collectively unique.

Progress in the identification process consists of growing awareness of the probabilities involved in making such assessments. Positive identification must be distinguished from putative, tentative, or possible identifications. Key to this distinction is assessment of the uniqueness of the features examined and the high bar required for positive identification (Stephan and Guyomarc'h 2015). Thoughtful research has contributed to realistic assessment of these issues, especially in radiographic analysis. Interpretation is influenced not only by the uniqueness of skeletal attributes but also by the highly variable quality of the images available for comparison, especially antemortem images of the once living individual.

Future progress in this area likely will focus on new studies of variation of the skeletal structures mostly commonly encountered in the positive identification process (Maxwell and Ross 2014; Stephan et al. 2014; Derrick et al. 2015). Automation and more rigorous statistical procedures will also likely impact procedures in positive ways (Lee et al. 2015; Stephan 2015).

1.11 Foul play

Forensic anthropologists routinely make unique contributions to evaluations of foul play involving skeletal remains. Although determination of cause and manner of death is a responsibility of forensic pathologists, anthropologists frequently present key evidence that contributes to such determinations (Fleischman 2015). Once alterations are detected, analysis must determine if they represent antemortem conditions that likely were not related to the death event, postmortem, and taphonomic processes or those that may be related to the death event (Cunha and Pinheiro 2009). Those possibly related to the death event are frequently described as being perimortem, indicating they were produced at or around the time of death (Loe 2009).

Considerable advancement has been sustained in this area through enhanced assessment of taphonomic factors (as previously outlined), better understanding of the evidence for bone remodeling suggestive of the antemortem condition, and studies of skeletal trauma (Rickman and Smith 2014; Beck et al. 2015). The trauma studies include more nuanced understanding of the bone fracture process and how the type of trauma can be determined from skeletal alterations (Love et al. 2015; Pinto et al. 2015; Wiersema et al. 2015). Also important are studies to help determine if fractures and evidence of various types of injury were sustained in the perimortem window or postmortem (Cappella et al. 2014; Báez-Molgado et al. 2015).

Experimental research likely will fuel future progress in this area. More knowledge is needed regarding additional factors that produce bone alterations and the impact of such postmortem conditions as thermal change, exposure to different environments and different rates and types of taphonomic processes (Dussault et al. 2014; Smith 2014; Robbins et al. 2015).

1.12 Certification

As in other areas of forensic science, individual certification represents an important issue. With growing numbers of professionals in the general field of anthropology attracted to forensic applications, it is important to reinforce standards of qualification. In North America, the American Board of Forensic Anthropology has offered certification to qualified anthropologists since 1977. Currently, certification is not limited to residents of North America but requires a doctorate degree relating to forensic anthropology and three years of experience in the field following receipt of the degree. Qualified applicants must also pass an examination administered by the ABFA. Since 1977, 111 individuals have been certified and 77 remain active in 2015.

Certification in forensic anthropology is also available in Latin America through the Asociación Latinoamericana de Antropología Forense. Qualified individuals also must pass an examination.

The United Kingdom offers certification in forensic anthropology through the Royal Anthropological Institute. The UK certification program recognizes three levels of expertise. Certification also is available through the Forensic Anthropology Society of Europe, a section of the International Academy of Legal Medicine. The FASE system recognizes two levels of expertise and also awards Honoris Causa certification to very experienced and established practitioners.

The certification programs previously described attempt in varying ways to credential qualified colleagues and provide the legal system some assurance that involved forensic anthropologists have the necessary skills and experience. These programs address the dual challenges of attempting to maintain high standards yet also recognize the highly variable backgrounds of those currently practicing in the field.

1.13 Conclusion

Forensic anthropology represents a robust and rapidly evolving field that embraces new research and experimentation. Central issues in the future likely will involve establishing probabilities associated with the many techniques utilized, expanded certification programs, laboratory accreditation, better understanding the varied impacts of global variation, and new applications.

Forensic anthropology continues to attract highly qualified students and professionals. They are welcome since they bring fresh perspective, new research ideas, and provide the numbers needed to address rapidly expanding applications. As with other areas of forensic science, forensic anthropology offers those involved an opportunity to use science to address key issues in contemporary society. These applications are likely to become more robust due to the high quality of new students entering this field.

Acknowledgments

The author would like to thank Madeleine Rosenstein of the George Washington University and Cassandra DeGaglia of the Smithsonian Institution for their assistance in the preparation of bibliographic materials.

References

Amores, A., Botella, M., and Alemán, I. (2014). Sexual dimorphism in the 7th cervical and 12th thoracic vertebrae from a Mediterranean population. *Journal of Forensic Sciences* 59 (2): 301–305.

Báez-Molgado, S., Bartelink, E., Jellema, L. et al. (2015). Classification of pelvic ring fractures in skeletonized human remains. *Journal of Forensic Sciences* 60 (S1): S171–S176.

Baker, L. (2009). Biomolecular applications. In: *Handbook of Forensic Anthropology and Archaeology* (ed. S. Blau and D.H. Ubelaker), 322–334. Walnut Creek, CA: Left Coast Press, Inc.

Beck, J., Ostericher, I., Sollish, G., and De Léon, J. (2015). Animal scavenging and scattering and the implications for documenting the deaths of undocumented border crossers in the Sonoran Desert. *Journal of Forensic Sciences* 60 (S1): S11–S20.

Boyd, K., Villa, C., and Lynnerup, N. (2015). The use of CT scans in estimating age at death by examining the extent of ectocranial suture closure. *Journal of Forensic Sciences* 60 (2): 363–369.

Brzobohatá, H., Krajíček, V., Horák, Z., and Velemínská, J. (2015). Sex classification using the three-dimensional tibia form or shape including population specificity approach. *Journal of Forensic Sciences* 60 (1): 29–40.

Cappella, A., Amadasi, A., Castoldi, E. et al. (2014). The difficult task of assessing perimortem and postmortem fractures on the skeleton: a blind text on 210 fractures of known origin. *Journal of Forensic Sciences* 59 (6): 1598–1601.

Cheetham, P.N. and Hanson, I. (2009). Excavation and recovery in forensic archaeological investigations. In: *Handbook of Forensic Anthropology and Archaeology* (ed. S. Blau and D.H. Ubelaker), 141–149. Walnut Creek, CA: Left Coast Press, Inc.

Cunha, E. and Pinheiro, J. (2009). Antemortem trauma. In: *Handbook of Forensic Anthropology and Archaeology* (ed. S. Blau and D.H. Ubelaker), 246–262. Walnut Creek, CA: Left Coast Press, Inc.

Dabbs, G.R. (2015). How should forensic anthropologists correct national weather service temperature data for use in estimating the postmortem interval? *Journal of Forensic Sciences* 60 (3): 581–587.

De Angelis, D., Mele, E., Gibelli, D. et al. (2015). The applicability of the Lamendin method to skeletal remains buried for a 16-year period: a cautionary note. *Journal of Forensic Sciences* 60 (S1): S177–S181.

Derrick, S.M., Raxter, M.H., Hipp, J.A. et al. (2015). Development of computer-assisted forensic radiographic identification method using the lateral cervical and lumbar spine. *Journal of Forensic Sciences* 60 (1): 5–12.

Dussault, M.C., Smith, M., and Osselton, D. (2014). Blast injury and the human skeleton: an important emerging aspect of conflict-related trauma. *Journal of Forensic Sciences* 59 (3): 606–612.

Fateh, E.E.A., Shirley, N.R., Jantz, R.L., and Mahfouz, M.R. (2014). Improving sex estimation from crania using a novel three-dimensional quantitative method. *Journal of Forensic Sciences* 59 (3): 590–600.

Fleischman, J.M. (2015). Radiographic identification using midline medical sternotomy wires. *Journal of Forensic Sciences* 60 (S1): S3–S10.

Forbes, S. and Nugent, K. (2009). Dating of anthropological skeletal remains of forensic interest. In: *Handbook of Forensic Anthropology and Archaeology* (ed. S. Blau and D.H. Ubelaker), 164–173. Walnut Creek, CA: Left Coast Press, Inc.

Guglich, E.A., Wilson, P.J., and White, B.N. (1994). Forensic application of repetitive DNA markers to the species identification of animal tissues. *Journal of Forensic Sciences* 39 (2): 353–361.

Hefner, J.T. and Ousley, S.D. (2014). Statistical classification methods for estimating ancestry using morphoscopic traits. *Journal of Forensic Sciences* 59 (4): 883–890.

Holland, T.D. and Connell, S.V. (2009). The search for and detection of human remains. In: *Handbook of Forensic Anthropology and Archaeology* (ed. S. Blau and D.H. Ubelaker), 129–140. Walnut Creek, CA: Left Coast Press, Inc.

Kanz, F., Reiter, C., and Risser, D.U. (2014). Citrate content of bone for time since death estimation: results from burials with different physical characteristics and known PMI. *Journal of Forensic Sciences* 59 (3): 613–620.

Klales, A.R. and Kenyhercz, M.W. (2015). Morphological assessment of ancestry using cranial macromorphoscopics. *Journal of Forensic Sciences* 60 (1): 13–20.

Lee, W.J., Wilkinson, C.M., Hwang, H.S., and Lee, S.M. (2015). Correlation between average tissue depth data and quantitative accuracy of forensic craniofacial reconstructions measured by geometric surface comparison method. *Journal of Forensic Sciences* 60 (3): 572–580.

Lesciotto, K.M. (2015). The impact of Daubert on the admissibility of forensic anthropology expert testimony. *Journal of Forensic Sciences* 60 (3): 549–555.

Loe, L. (2009). Perimortem trauma. In: *Handbook of Forensic Anthropology and Archaeology* (ed. S. Blau and D.H. Ubelaker), 263–283. Walnut Creek, CA: Left Coast Press, Inc.

Love, J.C., Derrick, S.M., Wiersema, J.M., and Peters, C. (2015). Microscopic saw mark analysis: an empirical approach. *Journal of Forensic Sciences* 60 (S1): S21–S26.

Maxwell, A.B. and Ross, A.H. (2014). A radiographic study on the utility of cranial vault outlines for positive identification. *Journal of Forensic Sciences* 59 (2): 314–318.

Mays, S. (2014). A test of recently devised method of estimating skeletal age at death using features of the adult acetabulum. *Journal of Forensic Sciences* 59 (1): 184–187.

Merritt, C.E. (2014). A test of Hartnett's revisions to the public symphysis and fourth rib methods on a modern sample. *Journal of Forensic Sciences* 59 (3): 703–711.

Michel, J., Paganelli, A., Varoquaux, A. et al. (2015). Determination of sex: interest of front sinus 3D reconstructions. *Journal of Forensic Sciences* 60 (2): 269–273.

Moraitis, K., Zorba, E., Eliopoulos, C., and Fox, S.C. (2014). A test of the revised auricular surface aging method on a modern European population. *Journal of Forensic Sciences* 59 (1): 188–194.

Mulhern, D.M. (2009). Differentiating human from nonhuman skeletal remains. In: *Handbook of Forensic Anthropology and Archaeology* (ed. S. Blau and D.H. Ubelaker), 153–163. Walnut Creek, CA: Left Coast Press, Inc.

Nawrocki, S.P. (2009). Forensic taphonomy. In: *Handbook of Forensic Anthropology and Archaeology* (ed. S. Blau and D.H. Ubelaker), 284–294. Walnut Creek, CA: Left Coast Press, Inc.

Ostrofsky, K.R. and Churchill, S.E. (2015). Sex determination by discriminant function analysis of lumbar vertebrae. *Journal of Forensic Sciences* 60 (1): 21–28.

Pilloud, M.A., Hefner, J.T., Hanihara, T., and Hayashi, A. (2014). The use of tooth crown measurements in the assessment of ancestry. *Journal of Forensic Sciences* 59 (6): 1493–1501.

Pinto, D.C., Love, J.C., Derrick, S.M. et al. (2015). A proposed scheme for classifying pediatric rib head fractures using case examples. *Journal of Forensic Sciences* 60 (1): 112–117.

Rickman, J.M. and Smith, M.J. (2014). Scanning electron microscope analysis of gunshot defects to bone: an underutilized source of information on ballistic trauma. *Journal of Forensic Sciences* 59 (6): 1473–1486.

Robbins, S.C., Fairgrieve, S.I., and Tracy, S.O. (2015). Interpreting the effects of burning on pre-incineration saw marks in bone. *Journal of Forensic Sciences* 60 (S1): S182–S187.

Roberts, L.G. and Dabbs, G.R. (2015). A taphonomic study exploring the differences in decomposition rate and manner between frozen and never frozen domestic pigs (*Sus scrofa*). *Journal of Forensic Sciences* 60 (3): 588–594.

Rogers, T.L. (2009). Skeletal age estimation. In: *Handbook of Forensic Anthropology and Archaeology* (ed. S. Blau and D.H. Ubelaker), 208–221. Walnut Creek, CA: Left Coast Press, Inc.

Sauer, N.J. and Wankmiller, J.W. (2009). The assessment of ancestry and the concept of race. In: *Handbook of Forensic Anthropology and Archaeology* (ed. S. Blau and D.H. Ubelaker), 187–200. Walnut Creek, CA: Left Coast Press, Inc.

Shirley, N.R. and Ramirez Montes, P.A. (2015). Age estimation in forensic anthropology: quantifications of observer error in phase versus component-based methods. *Journal of Forensic Sciences* 60 (1): 107–111.

Smith, A.C. (2014). The effects of sharp-force thoracic trauma on the rate and pattern of decomposition. *Journal of Forensic Sciences* 59 (2): 319–326.

Spradley, M.K., Anderson, B.E., and Tise, M.L. (2015). Postcranial sex estimation criteria for Mexican Hispanics. *Journal of Forensic Sciences* 60 (S1): S27–S31.

Steadman, D. (2013). The places we will go: paths forward in forensic anthropology. In: *Forensic Science: Current Issues, Future Directions* (ed. D.H. Ubelaker), 131–159. West Sussex: Wiley.

Stephan, C.N. (2015). Facial approximation – from facial reconstruction synonym to face prediction paradigm. *Journal of Forensic Sciences* 60 (3): 566–571.

Stephan, C.N. and Guyomarc'h, P. (2015). Qualification and perspective-induced shape change of clavicles at radiology and 3D scanning to assist human identification. *Journal of Forensic Sciences* 59 (2): 447–453.

Stephan, C.N., Amidan, B., Trease, H. et al. (2014). Morphometric comparison of clavicle outlines from 3D bone scans and 2D chest radiographs: a shortlisting tool to assist radiographic identification of human skeletons. *Journal of Forensic Sciences* 59 (2): 306–313.

Ubelaker, D.H. (2014a). Osteology reference collections. In: *Encyclopedia of Global Archaeology*, vol. 8 (ed. C. Smith), 5632–5641. New York, NY: Springer.

Ubelaker, D.H. (2014b). Radiocarbon analysis of human remains: a review of forensic application. *Journal of Forensic Sciences* 59 (6): 1466–1472.

Ubelaker, D.H., Ward, D.C., Braz, V.S., and Stewart, J. (2002). The use of SEM/EDS analysis to distinguish dental and osseous tissue from other materials. *Journal of Forensic Sciences* 47 (5): 940–943.

Ubelaker, D.H., Lowenstein, J.M., and Hood, D.G. (2004). Use of solid-phase double-antibody radioimmunoassay to identify species from small skeletal fragments. *Journal of Forensic Sciences* 49 (5): 924–929.

Ubelaker, D.H., Buchholz, B.A., and Stewart, J.E.B. (2006). Analysis of artificial radiocarbon in different skeletal and dental tissue types to evaluate date of death. *Journal of Forensic Sciences* 51 (3): 484–488.

Villa, C., Buckberry, J., Cattaneo, C. et al. (2015). Quantitative analysis of the morphological changes of the pubic symphyseal face and the auricular surface and implications for age at death estimation. *Journal of Forensic Sciences* 60 (3): 556–565.

Wescott, D.J. (2015). Sexual dimorphism in auricular surface projection and postauricular sulcus morphology. *Journal of Forensic Sciences* 60 (3): 679–685.

Wiersema, J.M., Derrick, S.M., Pinto, D.C. et al. (2015). Standardized descriptive method for the anthropological evaluation of pediatric skull fractures. *Journal of Forensic Sciences* 59 (6): 1487–1492.

Willey, P. (2009). Stature estimation. In: *Handbook of Forensic Anthropology and Archaeology* (ed. S. Blau and D.H. Ubelaker), 236–245. Walnut Creek, CA: Left Coast Press, Inc.

Wink, A.E. (2014). Pubic symphyseal age estimation from three-dimensional reconstructions of pelvic CT scans of live individuals. *Journal of Forensic Sciences* 59 (3): 696–702.

Young, A., Márquez-Grant, N., Stillman, R. et al. (2015). An investigation of red fox (*Vulpes vulpes*) and eurasian badger (*Meles meles*) scavenging, scattering, and removal of deer remains: forensic implications and applications. *Journal of Forensic Sciences* 60 (S1): S39–S55.

Zapico, S.C. and Ubelaker, D.H. (2013a). mtDNA mutations and their role in aging, diseases and forensic sciences. *Aging Diseases* 4 (6): 364–380.

Zapico, S.C. and Ubelaker, D.H. (2013b). Sex determination from dentin and pulp in a medicolegal context. *The Journal of the American Dental Association* 144 (12): 1379–1386.

Zimmerman, H.A., Schultz, J.J., and Sigmund, M.E. (2015). Preliminary validation of handheld X-ray fluorescence spectrometry: distinguishing osseous and dental tissue from nonbone material of similar chemical composition. *Journal of Forensic Sciences* 60 (2): 382–390.

CHAPTER 2

Some thoughts on the future challenges to criminalistics

Ronald L. Singer

Tarrant County Medical Examiner's District, Fort Worth, TX, USA

"May you live in interesting times."

(Origin disputed)

2.1 Introduction

The quote aforementioned is actually supposed to be a curse—a wish that your life be filled with the stresses and pressures of constant turmoil and of changes over which you have little control. The public's increased awareness of criminalistics, due to both positive (television, novels, and technological advances) and negative (highly publicized exonerations, the 2009 report of the National Academy of Science) pressures, has made these times very "interesting" for the field of criminalistics, and it promises to continue to be interesting for some time to come. Not only have the times become interesting for those working in the field but these pressures, and the field's reaction to them, have also attracted the attention of people who may not be scientists, but who are in positions that enable them to add to these pressures through legislation, the media, or other outlets.

"Criminalistics" is generally defined as the evaluation of physical evidence by the application of the laws of natural science. It includes the following:

The Future of Forensic Science, First Edition. Edited by Daniel A. Martell.
© 2019 John Wiley & Sons Ltd. Published 2019 by John Wiley & Sons Ltd.

1. *Firearm/toolmark examination*, which includes the examination of firearms to determine their condition, a comparison of fired ammunition components to test fired material from known firearms, serial number restoration, distance determination, and other studies relating to firearms and ammunition components;

2. *Forensic biology* that includes the identification of biologic fluids (serology) and DNA analysis;

3. *Trace evidence*, which is the evaluation and identification of materials that because of their size or weight can be easily transferred from one object or individual to another, and includes materials such as hair, fibers, glass, paint, gunshot residue as well as the evaluation of shoe prints and tire tracks;

4. *Drug chemistry*, which is the analysis of pills, powders, liquids, etc. for the presence of controlled dangerous substances; and it may also include, depending on who you ask;

5. *Fingerprint examination*, which includes the visualization and comparison of fingerprints; and

6. *Forensic photography*, which involves the photography of physical evidence using specialized techniques as well as the evaluation of photographs and other photographic materials for authenticity, source, etc.

Criminalistics is being challenged by a number of factors. Not all are necessarily bad, but all will require some adjustments on the part of the scientists performing the work, and the agencies and managers who are overseeing the processes. In the paragraphs that follow, some of these issues will be explored.

2.2 Technological advances

2.2.1 Computers, software, and databases

Computers are now integral parts of highly sophisticated analytical tools and are serving as repositories for information that can be searched, sorted, and queried much more rapidly than ever before. Technological advances and the increased reliance on computer-driven systems and databases will continue to reduce the time required for analytical processes, make them more specific, and even allow procedures to be handled at the crime scene as opposed to the laboratory. Databases now allow the accumulation of information that can be rapidly searched, providing not only the ability to develop statistical models for many types of evidence but also to make preliminary comparisons electronically. Currently, local and national databases exist that accumulate and store DNA profiles, fingerprints, firearms rifling characteristics, information about the surface details of fired bullets and cartridge cases, chemical profiles of paint, information about explosive and flammable compounds, the sole patterns on shoes, tread patterns on tires, the list goes on and on and is increasing daily. Computers and other digital devices such as cell phones, tablets, and the data stored on them are also becoming increasingly important as items of evidence.

2.2.2 DNA

In the last 25 years, DNA has replaced fingerprints as the "gold standard" in identification. As DNA technology becomes more advanced, probative information will be obtained from smaller and smaller samples; we will be able to predict physical features based on the DNA profile developed from unknown biological material left at crime scenes; and software programs will allow the interpretation of more and more complex mixtures. With these advances will come challenges that will have to be addressed. As the size of DNA databases grow, the potential for unrelated matching profiles existing also grows, making it necessary to add additional alleles to the DNA profiles generated. The interpretation of mixtures, particularly ones that contain profiles in varying concentrations will become more reliant on software programs rather than manual calculations. Finally, as analytical equipment becomes smaller and more portable, scientists may have to shift their focus from the bench to the preparation and monitoring of protocols for methods actually applied in the field by nonscientists.

2.2.3 Impression evidence

Impression evidence includes the examination and comparison of markings left by the interaction of firearms with the ammunition fired from them, the comparison of the design features and incidental markings left by wear on shoe soles and tires, and the evaluation and comparison of fingerprints. In the case of firearms and toolmarks, this examination has traditionally been based on a side-by-side visual comparison of material recovered from a crime scene (the "unknown") to exemplars produced by the suspect firearm, screwdriver, crowbar, or other tool (the "known") in an attempt to determine if there is sufficient correspondence between the random markings on the surfaces of the items to conclude that they were made by the same firearm or tool. This comparison is conducted using a comparison microscope, which consists of two microscopes linked together by an optical bridge, allowing for the simultaneous examination of the surfaces of both the known and unknown samples. The final determination as to whether or not the known firearm or tool was the source of the markings on the unknown evidence is made based on the experience and training of the examiner. Fingerprint, shoeprint, and tire mark comparisons are conducted in a like fashion, looking for a correspondence between random characteristics in the ridge detail of the skin of the fingers ("minutiae") or random markings left behind on shoe soles or tires as a result of the wear of that object ("wear marks"). This is accomplished either with the aid of some magnification or with the naked eye. Computer-assisted evaluation of these surfaces is reducing the subjectivity of these types of analyses; as the software driving these computers becomes more sophisticated, forensic scientists will at last be able to assign statistical relevance to the markings that are observed. This will require a change in the manner in which testimony in these areas is offered; no longer will a forensic scientist be able to emphatically state that a fingerprint was made by one particular individual to the exclusion of all others, that a particular ammunition component was fired from a single firearm, or that an impression left at a scene was made by a particular shoe or tire. Rather, testimony in these areas will become more like that expected in DNA cases, with some statistical relevance assigned to the correspondences observed.

2.2.4 Instrumentation

As instrumentation becomes more sophisticated, it becomes smaller, it provides more information, it becomes faster, and at least in the beginning, it becomes more expensive. Up-front and continuing maintenance costs aside, major advances in the precision and accuracy of instrumentation will require more advanced training on the part of the forensic scientists expected to use the equipment, which can create a strain on the staffing of the laboratory and requires additional budgeting to provide for the cost of the training. In addition, as instruments become smaller and more portable, they will be adapted for use at the scene rather than in the laboratory. This will cause a change in the forensic scientist's basic role from production at the bench to supervision, certification, and training of nonscientists who will be using the equipment at the scene.

2.3 Quality issues

2.3.1 NAS Report

In 2005, the United States Congress directed the National Academy of Sciences to conduct a study on the state of forensic science in the United States. The report of that study, issued in February 2009, created ripples throughout the forensic science community, particularly in the area of criminalistics. Discussions began almost immediately in Congress regarding the establishment of federal standards and other requirements for forensic scientists, and various committees were formed to expedite the process. The inevitable outcome of this process will be the passing of federal legislation; how rigorous the requirements are will be dependent on the input from these various committees, but they will surely involve mandatory laboratory accreditation and individual certification, as well as the establishment of standard methods of analysis, or "best practices." In order to ensure that these changes occur, additional funding will have to be made available, most likely from federal grants. While additional funding for laboratories and for the continuing education necessary to prepare for certification is always welcome, the question inevitably arises regarding where this money will come from once federal funding ceases. In addition, some states, such as Texas, have established oversight bodies of their own. Depending on the authority afforded to these bodies by their state legislatures, additional requirements may be imposed on forensic laboratories. These requirements may include licensing, additional accreditation criteria, and additional reporting requirements. Laboratories and laboratory personnel will have to adjust to new levels of scrutiny, often by boards or commissions whose membership is beyond their control. An unintended consequence of this additional layer of oversight may very well be a need to increase administrative and clerical staff in order to keep up with added record-keeping functions, increasing the financial burden on the laboratory's parent agency. The NAS Report was also critical of the fact that most forensic laboratories are closely associated with law enforcement agencies. We have already seen the beginnings of a shift away from forensic laboratories being a part of law enforcement, with the establishment of independent, board-controlled public laboratories, laboratories established as part of medical examiner's offices, and private laboratories that contract with various law enforcement agencies to provide forensic services. This trend will change the basic relationship between the laboratory and its clients; the laboratory will no longer serve a single entity (the law enforcement agency of which it was once a part) but rather will be serving a varied clientele, including law enforcement, prosecutors, defense attorneys, the judiciary, and even individuals. While quality of service and accountability to their clients will continue to dominate the laboratory's processes, there will be considerably more scrutiny from outside sources, and customer satisfaction will become a major concern.

2.4   Financial burdens

As previously mentioned, change inevitably costs money. Obtaining, and keeping, this additional funding will become a major challenge for forensic laboratories; this will lead to hard decisions not only about the source of this funding but also how to make the best use of whatever funding becomes available. Since the vast majority of public crime laboratories are part of some larger agency, care must be taken to ensure that any additional funding coming from the parent agency not be a one-time appropriation with no long-term support. Commitments of this sort are very hard to come by, as priorities tend to shift over time. It will become essential that laboratories devise methods that will either ensure continued funding, which will be difficult at best, or find ways to derive the most benefit from the funds available to them, which is a much more likely scenario. Among the choices available to laboratories are the following:

2.4.1 Seeking additional sources of grant funding

Although grants suffer from the same issues mentioned previously regarding agency funding, that is the lack of consistency in available funding and the inevitable dependency on the financial and political fortunes of those distributing the funds, grants can be useful to fill gaps that may occur in other, more permanent sources of funding. The tendency has been to rely on grants made available by the Federal government, or through State Criminal Justice granting agencies. As these funds become less available, other sources, such as private foundations or research institutions, will have to be explored. However, because of the inconsistencies inherent in funding of this sort, grants can never be the complete answer to increasing financial burdens and should never be relied upon for long-term funding.

2.4.2 Staffing

As processes become more complicated, both from a technical as well as administrative standpoint, increasing demands will be placed on individual forensic scientists. More critical processes, such as the interpretation of mixtures of DNA profiles, will require additional training and education. Even as newer instrumentation reduces the actual analytical time, added layers of technical and administrative review and increased process control measures will in many cases actually lengthen the average turnaround time required for each case. The trend toward specialization among forensic scientists will continue, leading to a need to increase staffing. If funding is not available, increasing staff will be problematic; decisions will have to be made regarding the best use of the staff levels available. This may lead to a reduction in the services offered, allowing administrations to concentrate on services that are of the most benefit to the laboratory's particular clientele. However, many of these services, even though they may not provide data as specific as DNA may, still provide valuable investigative information and to abandon them would create a gap in the scientific support of the investigation of criminal activity. Consequently, reallocation of staffing needs to be combined with other cost-saving measures in order to maximize the effectiveness of the resources available.

2.4.3 Regionalization

One possible solution to the problem mentioned previously is the regionalization of some services. If a state is serviced by a system of regional state laboratories, rather than offer a complete list of services at every laboratory, it may be possible to offer some services such as certain types of trace analyses in only one of the laboratories. Cases would then be sent there from all locations for evaluation. Although this will reduce the staffing and equipment needs overall, the trade-off would be an increase in the length of time required to get information back to the submitting agency. It could also increase the cost of travel for analysts required to testify in trials. However, substantial savings could still be made even if certain services were eliminated in half the laboratories in the system. On a local basis, the same system could be established if local laboratories are close enough together or even serve overlapping jurisdictions. Laboratories could agree to make specific services available to nearby laboratories while obtaining other services from them. On the negative side, agreements such as this will usually involve negotiations between the parent agencies and the formulating and signing of memoranda of understanding ("MOU's"). These can take long periods of time to work out and often lead to complications. On the other hand, informal agreements made between laboratories can often help relieve temporary backlogs and foster further cooperative efforts.

2.4.4 Consolidation

A more drastic step would involve the consolidation of two or more laboratories operating in nearby or overlapping areas into a single laboratory. Consolidation has several advantages—participating agencies contribute financial support to a single laboratory as opposed to two or more individual laboratories; a single set of necessary equipment is needed rather than equipping two or more laboratories with the same or similar equipment; manpower needs are cut, and only one physical plant needs to be maintained. The participating agencies could end up with a single laboratory with capabilities far greater than any of the single laboratories it replaces, with substantial savings in costs to each of the participants.

Consolidation is not without its challenges, however. A major issue bound to arise is how control is going to be exercised over the facility. If a larger laboratory is taking over the functions of other smaller laboratories, the larger laboratory's parent agency will generally continue to assert ultimate control over the resulting facility; however, if none of the laboratories joining together is larger or offers more services, a conflict over ultimate control could result. Where will this "new" laboratory be located? Who do the forensic scientists in the laboratory work for, and will they be receiving benefits comparable to the ones they were receiving before the consolidation? All these questions, and more, would need to be carefully considered before any type of consolidation can take place. On an individual basis, the forensic scientists working in the facility may have to adjust to new management styles, new policies and procedures, and new coworkers.

2.4.5 Cost recovery

Another means of supporting laboratory functions is through some method of cost recovery. In some cases, regionalization, consolidation, or even simply funding current operations may still have to be paid for by instituting a charge for the services provided. If a laboratory is within a larger public agency and is only serving that agency, the costs of doing business are by necessity absorbed by the parent agency. How much money is available is a factor of the agency's overall financial health, the laboratory's position within the departmental hierarchy, the administration's attitude regarding the usefulness of the laboratory, and a host of other issues. However, if the forensic laboratory accepts cases from agencies besides the parent agency, the laboratory may want to consider charging those other agencies utilizing the service. Since public agencies are by their nature non-profitable, the goal of instituting a fee schedule is simply to recover the actual costs of providing the service; however, the fees collected relieve some of the costs that would otherwise be paid by the parent agency. The saved money could be used to enhance the quality of the laboratory or could be added back to the parent agency's general fund for use in other projects.

Other cost recovery methods that may be considered are the attachment of fees dedicated to the forensic laboratory to court costs imposed on guilty pleas and convictions and contracts with agencies based on population or overall usage rather than on a per case or per analysis basis. Negotiating and maintaining agreements such as this can be complicated and burdensome, and once again, the forensic laboratory is at the mercy of the financial and political fortunes of the source of the funding.

2.4.6 Privatization

Rather than totally dropping services, or increasing the time required to work and report cases to unacceptable levels, forensic laboratories might also consider outsourcing some of the work to independent private laboratories. Because laboratories can use the bidding process to choose an outside laboratory, and because the total cost can be spread between the laboratory (for the analytical work) and the District Attorney's Office (for the testimony; it also saves the laboratory money spent in lost analysis time when the forensic scientist is out of the laboratory testifying), outsourcing can actually save a laboratory money. What is lost is the parent agency and/or the forensic laboratory's control over the processes once the samples leave their hands. In addition, many District Attorneys oppose outsourcing because of the added cost to them. Also, when the private laboratory is located in another city or another state, there could be a breakdown of the one-on-one relationship that develops between the forensic laboratory and their clients.

Lack of funding or other financial burdens pose a major challenge to criminalistics; however, it should never be used as an excuse for poor performance. The real challenge facing the field is how the resources that are available are going to be used to the maximum benefit by the laboratories while still maintaining a high level of reliability and quality in the work that they do.

Criminalistics indeed lives in "interesting times." However, since 2009 and before, the men and women involved in the research, analysis, and administration of the science have worked diligently to meet the pressures and challenges that the field has presented, and it is clear that they will continue to meet, and overcome, those challenges.

Acknowledgments

This is an expansion of a presentation made at the Interdisciplinary Symposium of the American Academy of Forensic Sciences at its 67th annual scientific meeting, February 2015, Orlando, Florida. The author wishes to thank AAFS Past Presidents Douglas M. Lucas (1972–1973), Richard S. Frank (1988–1989), Barry A.J. Fisher (1998–1999), and Joseph P. Bono (2010–2011) for their contributions to the ideas and content of the original presentation, which formed the basis for this effort.

References

National Research Council, Strengthening Forensic Science in the United States: A Path Forward. National Academies Press, Document Number 2280901, August 2009. Available at www.nap.edu/catalog/12588.htm

Texas Forensic Science Commission, www.txcourts.gov/fsc/about-us/

Houston Forensic Science Center, www.houstonforensicscience.org/

CHAPTER 3

Digital and multimedia sciences

Zeno Geradts

Department of Digital and Biometric Traces, Netherlands Forensic Institute,
The Netherlands
Chair Forensic Data Science, Informatics Institute, University of Amsterdam,
The Netherlands

3.1 Introduction

Over the last decades, the amount of digital storage and devices grew exponentially. Most citizens, and criminals, now own devices like smart phones and computers and use them almost continuously for their profession and in their private lives. In addition, CCTV cameras observe people in public spaces and private companies. As a result, such devices often carry huge amounts of data on them. This data might be information from databases, multimedia information such as recorded video and audio, interaction and download logs, mobility data, location data, or links to digital information stored somewhere on the Internet and linked to various social networks. This influx of digital data has a tremendous impact on the field of forensics and is leading to new research challenges. In this chapter, an overview is given on the selection of developments; however, due to the rapidly changing field and the wide range of topics this overview is not complete.

The Future of Forensic Science, First Edition. Edited by Daniel A. Martell.
© 2019 John Wiley & Sons Ltd. Published 2019 by John Wiley & Sons Ltd.

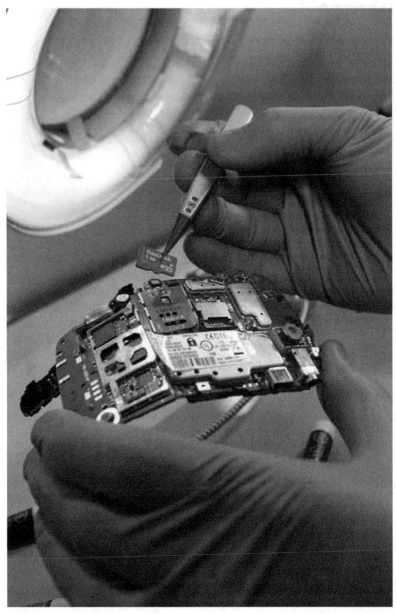

Forensic Investigation of a mobile phone. Source: Netherlands Forensic Institute.

3.2 History

Carrie Whitcomb, past vice president of the American Academy of Forensic Sciences (AAFS), described that already in 1984, the FBI started with a unit of computer evidence (Whitcomb 2002). In 1995, according to a survey by the US Secret Service (USSS), it appeared that 48% of the agencies had a computer crime lab active in the United States.

The issue of standardization was already discussed earlier. In 1991, a group of six international law enforcement agencies had a meeting with several US federal law enforcement agencies in Charleston, South Carolina, to discuss computer forensic science and the need for standardized approach to examinations. In 1993, the FBI hosted an International Law Enforcement Conference on Computer Evidence that was attended by 70 representatives of various US federal, state, and local law enforcement agencies. The participants agreed that standards for computer forensic science were needed.

A similar conference was organized in Baltimore, Maryland, in 1995, Australia in 1996, and the Netherlands in 1997, and resulted in the formation of the International Organization on Computer Evidence (IOCE). The IOCE seized to exist in 2010 after the last meeting was organized in Tokyo, Japan.

In Europe, ENFSI Started the Forensic IT Working group in 1997 in Prague, Czech Republic, which also had good connections with the IOCE and was also involved in writing several best practice guides.

In the United States on 17 June 1998, the Technical Working Group Digital Evidence (TWGDE) held their first meeting. Mark Pollitt, Special Agent, FBI, was elected Chair and Carrie Morgan Whitcomb, Manager, Forensic Services, US Postal Inspection Service was elected Co-Chair. Several federal forensic laboratories were represented including the Bureau of Alcohol, Tobacco, and Firearms (ATF), US Customs, the Drug Enforcement Administration (DEA), FBI, Immigration and Naturalization Service (INS), Internal Revenue Service (IRS), National Aeronautics and Space Administration (NASA), USSS, and the US Postal Inspection Service. The working group met monthly to prepare organizational procedures and develop relevant documents.

Later on the group was renamed to Scientific Working Group of Digital Evidence.[1] The Scientific Working group of Image Technology was split off this group and developed many best practice guides until 2015 after NIST launched the Organization of Scientific Area Committees (OSACs). At first, digital evidence was not seen as a separate group; however, in 2015, it was decided that digital evidence should be included in Digital/Multimedia Scientific Area Committee.

In 2002, Carrie Whitcomb gave a presentation for the board of the AAFS to emphasize the need for digital forensic science at the AAFS. Digital Evidence would be formed in the General Section as well as the Engineering Section. The Section Digital and Multimedia Sciences are the newest section within the AAFS and are founded in 2008 (Popejoy 2015). Digital devices, such as smart phones, computers, and digital electronics are common items and are almost everywhere since electronics are included in cars, medical devices, and many domestic equipment. From these devices, digital evidence can be extracted, which can be important in court. Also the multimedia side is expanding rapidly with cameras everywhere as well as the audio and speech that is combined with this.

Within the section, in a digital and multimedia examination might address some of the following questions.[2]

- What files have been deleted from the digital device?
- What other digital devices have been connected to this system?
- Was this system attacked or modified by someone over the network?
- Can a remote system or user be located or identified?
- What sites on the Internet were visited by this system?
- Was this audio recording altered?
- Can this video recording be enhanced to help identify someone?
- Can the physical characteristics of an object in a photograph be determined?
- Can individuals an offender targeted or victimized be determined?
- Can unknown victims be located or identified based on phone number, email, etc.?

---

[1] https://www.swgde.org
[2] http://old.aafs.org/students/student-career/digital-multimedia-sciences (accessed on 29 December 2015).

- Can patterns of offender activity related to the investigation be reconstructed?

3.3   Digital evidence

If we look into the digital competencies of forensic institutes,[3] most of them will focus on digital traces, the data, and the metadata. The top three kind of cases are child abuse, murder, and fraud investigations, and the top three investigation are mobile phones, storage devices, and data analysis.

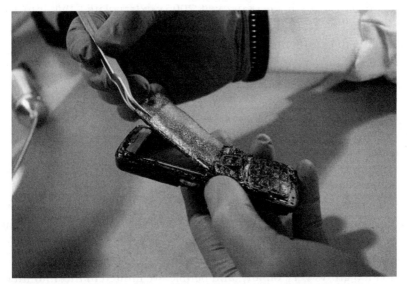

Investigating a burned phone. Source: Netherlands Forensic Institute.

Data that comes in from many sources, ranging from personal computers, backup tapes, lawful interception, smart phones, and many new devices were cameras and sensors are stored such as the drones. The development of new devices is very rapidly, so it is nearly impossible to be prepared for all new devices, so often research is needed to add the device to a knowledge database.

---

[3] Inaugural speech on Extracting evidence from Big Multimedia Data, University of Amsterdam, 2015, www.oratiereeks.nl/upload/pdf/PDF-2776weboratie_Geradts_-_DEF.pdf.

An issue with digital devices is that there exist many formats how the data is stored on the device and each day new formats become available. With over one million apps in the app stores, it is not easy to cover these all, and often with new updates of the software new storage formats are used. For this reason, it is important to have databases of tools and libraries of formats. In case this is not possible, the forensic investigator has to do reverse engineering, which can be time-consuming.

The amount of data is growing rapidly in the world, as well as the processing power. Raymond Kurzweil, in his book about the rate of growth of computing power he compared computational power. Using data on past growth he (Kurzweil 2005) extrapolated this into the future. He helped to make the rate of growth real to those not used to dealing in exponentials with the following:

- *In 2000, $1000 could buy a computer that had the computational power of an insect.*
- *In 2010, $1000 could buy a computer that had the computational power of a mouse.*
- *In 2020, $1000 could buy a computer that had the computational power of a human brain.*

The amount of different devices connected to the Internet is also thought to grow to 20 billion of devices in three years.

The amount of data (Zuech et al. 2015) is not the main issue always in forensic big data analytics. One of the issues with big data is the impossibility to process it with standard software in a timely manner. For images, these issues arise very soon since the amount of images and video grows very rapidly, and people are limited in the amount of images and hours of video they can process. Big data also means the amount of data, which can easily grow to 10 PB if we would collect all digital data confiscated by the police in 2015. Eight Terabyte is which is now often seen in practice, all of this data results in 40 km of trucks filled with paper if printed double-sided. However, at the same time, it is only 1600 h of HD video.

In the past (Nikkel 2014), there were many digital evidence systems developed on a standalone computer. The limitation is that the digital investigator has to search for keywords and with this iterative process with the tactical investigator, it might take months.

For new systems, the three implementations of security, privacy, and transparency are the main cornerstones of the system (Kloosterman et al. 2015). Security by design is important since one does not want to leak data, and not that data can be modified by other parties or the system administrators. The data as imaged by the police from the devices should remain intact. Also when examining the system, it is important that viruses and other malware that are examined do not infect the systems. Privacy (Dehghantanha and Franke 2014) is important since we see the amount of private data grows rapidly. Perhaps not all users realize how much information is stored on them concerning location by use of GPS and other location information in smart phones in combination with all the multimedia data that is stored on the device. Also often this is information shared with online cloud systems in often other countries. The advantage is that the data becomes available after a few hours (Geradts and Franke 2015) and the analyst and the tactical investigator can search through the data. With this method, the examination time can be reduced from months to the first results which become available in the first few hours after a crime happened.

More intelligent pattern recognition systems are needed, and images and video should be indexed. Validation of software remains important, however, as we can see is often not easy to do. Within the European Network of Forensic Institutes (Geradts 2011), a new best practice manual on digital evidence is published that also describes how to test the software and is also an effort to try to standardize and prevent.

Much efforts are given within the forensic community in the quality assurance. Validation and reporting the uncertainty in the interpretation of the evidence are important solutions for this.

3.4   Damaged (mobile) devices

In practice, also mobile devices are damaged due to thermal, radiation, mechanical impact, ballistics, or liquid. The field of recovering data is expanding now, with certain procedures to examine the memory chips of the devices and extracting data from them. In these cases, reconstruction of data and data carving is important, and best practice manuals are in preparation (Casey 2011; Scientific Working Group for Digital Evidence 2014).

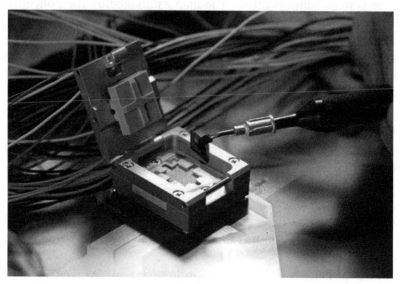

Chip extraction of a mobile phone. Source: Netherlands Forensic Institute.

3.5 Multimedia

The word "Multimedia" (Manjunath et al. 2002) has many meanings and often includes a combination of text, audio, still images, animation, location, and video. All these features combined result in a data analytics. When searching through data, often the combination of images, text, and location information is important to find information on when a certain image has been made and where it is having been made. Of course, within forensic science, one has to be aware that digital information can easily be altered, and this is sometimes a question from the court if the data has been tampered with. This is also called image forensics in literature. There exist several methods to automate this; however, for court cases, one should examine it manually since automated methods will contain falls hits. However, these can assist and reduce the time of investigation. It is advised to follow the best practice manuals, for example from the European Network of Forensic Science Institute (ENFSI) working groups and the Scientific Working groups for Image Technology and Digital Evidence to verify this.

3.5.1 Deep learning (Hinton et al. 2006)

In the 1990s neural networks (Geradts and Keijzer 1996) were already used for facial comparison and shoeprint comparisons. In the meantime, the computing power also of Graphical Processing Units (GPUs) expanded very much, so deep learning with more layers of a neural network was feasible. The algorithms for facial comparison and object recognition have improved for good quality images and are now used by law enforcement agencies.

The issue with humans (Beck et al. 2014) is that we have a very good vision system; however, we are not very good in bulk processing of thousands of hours of video. The computer is better in processing large amounts of images.

Current developments in (GPUs) make it possible to use more layers in a neural network for learning. This works well for good quality images, however, for most forensic images, it is still a challenge to the quality.

For facial comparison, the Facial Identification Scientific Working Group has written many best practice manuals,[4] also for automated system. They recommend certain education as well as a feature list that should be used in a forensic facial comparison.

Within multimedia forensics, recovery of damaged data is important (Grigoras 2010). Sometimes files are partly deleted and video and audio has to be recovered. Also a question that arises is the integrity and reliability of the evidence.

In questions like this if there has been tampering with the image (Mishra and Adhikary 2013) or the audio (Koenig and Lacey 2012), several approaches have been made to automatically detect this. However, once a method for detection is known, algorithm developers (Böhme and Kirchner 2013) might circumvent those, and also approaches are based on statistical approaches. In some images, it is

---

[4] https://www.fiswg.org/index

easy to prove they have been tampered with, especially if the source material is available. However, proving that the image has not been tampered with can be more difficult or even impossible.

Methods to estimate the time of a recording based on variations in the Electric Network Frequency (ENF) (Grigoras 2007; Huijbregtse and Geradts 2009) in an audio signal have reported to be used in court. Also the use of camera identification by using Photo Response Non Uniformity (PRNU) (van Houten et al. 2011) is also more widely used to prove that a certain image or a video has been recorded with a specific camera or mobile phone.

3.5.2   Camera identification

One research topic that had much interest is the camera identification (Lukas et al. 2006). The camera identification or Pixel Response Nonuniformity is to find a link between a camera and an image. Due to imperfections during the fabrication of the image sensors, this is a kind of pattern in images that is normally not visible with the human eye. By using an algorithm to filter this pattern out of a sequence of images or an image, the computer can fill a database of patterns.

By using a correlation method of these patterns, one can sometimes with a high likelihood ratio determine that the image has been made with a specific sensor. Validation in casework remains important, and procedures for using this in case reports are available.

This method can also be used for video (Chuang et al. 2011), and for casework, one can, for instance find a link between a camera found at a suspect and child pornography images. Also in other crime such as homicides this appeared to work as evidence to find a link between a suspect and a person that has been killed.

Even more one can also find relations between images if the camera is not in possession, as we can see with child pornography databases (Gisolf et al. 2013). One issue is that comparing all these patterns is time-consuming. So several approaches have been taken to limit the computation time.

In the past, we developed several proficiency tests for different labs within the ENFSI framework to answer these questions for a closed sets of cameras based on the noise patterns. In these proficiency tests, all labs have the right results on the comparison.

The method also appears to work with social networks such as YouTube and Facebook (Karaküçük et al. 2015), however, recently, it appears that the PRNU signal seems to be filtered out of the information.

3.5.3   Other biometrics

In child pornography cases, often the face is not visible. In this case, we might do a forensic comparison of hands (Slot and Geradts 2014), feet, and other body parts. These are conducted in a similar way as the facial comparison with three examiners comparing those independently from each other.

Soft biometrics is still in research phase; however, they are sometimes used as evidence in court.

3.6   Wearables and quantified self

A large range of wearables (Lillis et al. 2016) is available, ranging from virtual 3D glasses, to watches and health devices. The wearables are often on a person for a long time, and streaming photos and video to cloud systems is often combined. Also much of the location information and what kind of actions someone did at a given time is stored.

With the quantified self, we see that also heartbeat, breath patterns, blood pressure, walking, on a bicycle, and other actions are collected that can also be helpful in a forensic investigation. The amount of data that people produce is growing, and of course, a question remains if all this data can be used for forensic purposes based on privacy and security of the systems. They might even assist in investigations of the time of death.

3.7   Drones

The amount of drones (Horsman 2016) sold is increasing rapidly. These devices are important and challenges exist on what data can be taken from them. They can be also used for criminal acts, like attacking persons or dropping objects and intervene with regular air traffic.

For that reason, also data from these devices is important to collect in combination with time, date, and extracting information from the owner of the device. The drones are becoming much easier to use, since some of them have a follow-me option so one does not have to control it anymore.

3.8 Sensors

Sensors (Furner et al. 2015) on mobile devices are becoming much cheaper, as we can, for example see on the infrared sensors on mobile phones that are integrated easily on a phone for a few hundred euros instead of the thousands of euros they costed in the past. We also see that 3D imaging is getting cheaper nowadays, and the time is nearby that this is also integrated in smart phones.

3.9 Geo satellites

The development of higher-resolution satellite imaging systems (Sansurooah and Keane 2015), which in future make maps from the country every few days, can be useful for investigation. The combination of all images including the geo satellites with the information of location can be very important in digital evidence; however, investigators should be aware that uncertainty of location information and synchronization of time still remains an issue.

3.10 Disasters/large scale incidents

If there are large-scale incidents (Quintana et al. 2015) and disasters, we see that many images and videos are collected from devices and persons that are in the neighborhood of the accident. All these images and videos combined with digital data and other forensic information can lead to evidence in court.

3.11   Quality assurance

The Scientific Working groups of Digital Evidence and Image Technologies (SWGIT Milliet et al. 2014 and SWGDE Pollitt and Craiger 2014) have developed important best practice guides. Also several ANSI-standards have been developed or are in development. In the last few years, several guidelines have been published by ISO,[5] on handling digital evidence and the analysis and interpretation of digital evidence. The new OSACs (Butler 2014) on Digital and Multimedia are the following:
- Digital evidence
- Facial identification
- Speaker recognition and
- Video and Imaging Technology and Analysis.

These OSACS are considered important steps to improve the quality of the evidence for the future.

3.12   Challenges

For critical systems, such as banking systems and real-time information systems, it is important to look how to investigate these. Shutting down those systems can lead to a huge financial impact, and copying all the data might be nonproportional. Often, this can be solved by doing a live forensics investigation (Rahman and Khan 2015).

Also there are many issues with virtualization or storage, network, and servers in the cloud (Martini and Choo 2014). Questions on where the data resides, whose jurisdiction they are, and the owners of the information are important to answer. There are several challenges in cloud computing, since one has to rely on the cloud provider to provide all the evidence and that it also can be used in court. In court cases until now, there have been discussions on the reliability of the time stamps (Dykstra and Sherman 2012).

Furthermore, many criminals are aware that data is used in court cases (Dalziel 2014). For this reason, they will often use strong

---

[5] ISO/IEC 27037:2012; ISO/IEC 27042:2015.

encryption and one-time use devices to shield their identity and the information that they store. Also secure cloud computing networks such as Tornets are commonly used, and sometimes this is referred to as the dark web, though the users of Tor can also be legitimate.

One of the issues is that the amount of data is growing exponentially and the budgets of the forensic laboratories are not. It is not easy to keep up to date in methods and new technology that is available, and also it is a challenge to keep the employees, since the amount of students educated in International Criminal Tribunal (ICT) is still low (Siiman et al. 2014).

Other issues are that the interpretation of the digital and multimedia evidence is not always easy. The forensic scientist should be aware that complicated and new methods have to be explained in court. This means that preventing miscommunication as well as bias in the examination should be taken care of.

As digital technology is used by more people and more broadly (Bendovschi 2015), it is expected that cybercrime has much more impact on society. For international exchange, it is important that methods are exchanged internationally and public–private collaboration is needed to keep track with new developments.

References

Beck, J., Hope, B., and Rosenfeld, A. (eds.) (2014). *Human and Machine Vision*, vol. 8. Academic Press.

Bendovschi, A. (2015). Cyber-attacks-trends, patterns and security counter-measures. *Procedia Economics and Finance* 28: 24–31.

Böhme, R. and Kirchner, M. (2013). Counter-forensics: attacking image forensics. In: Sencar H., Memon N. (eds) *Digital Image Forensics*, 327–366. New York: Springer.

Butler, J.M. (2014). The national commission on forensic science and the Organization of Scientific Area Committees. In: *Proceedings of the International Symposium on Human Identification*. http://www.promega.com/products/pm/genetic-identity/ishi-conference-proceedings/25th-ishi-oral-presentations.

Casey, E. (2011). *Digital Evidence and Computer Crime: Forensic Science, Computers, and the Internet*. Academic Press.

Chuang, W.-H., Su, H., and Wu, M. (2011). Exploring compression effects for improved source camera identification using strongly compressed video. In: *2011 18th IEEE International Conference on Image Processing (ICIP)*. IEEE.

Dalziel, H. (2014). *Introduction to US Cybersecurity Careers.* Syngress.

Dehghantanha, A. and Franke, K. (2014). Privacy-respecting digital investigation. In: *2014 Twelfth Annual International Conference on Privacy, Security and Trust (PST).* IEEE.

Dykstra, J. and Sherman, A.T. (2012). Acquiring forensic evidence from infrastructure-as-a-service cloud computing: exploring and evaluating tools, trust, and techniques. *Digital Investigation* 9: S90–S98.

Furner, C.P., Racherla, P., and Babb, J.S. (2015). What we know and do not know about mobile app usage and stickiness: a research agenda. *International Journal of E-Services and Mobile Applications (IJESMA)* 7 (3): 48–69.

Geradts, Z. (2011). ENFSI forensic IT working group. *Digital Investigation* 8 (2): 94–95.

Geradts, Z.J. and Franke, K. (2015). Editorial for big data issue. *Digital Investigation* 15: 18–19.

Geradts, Z. and Keijzer, J. (1996). The image-database REBEZO for shoeprints with developments on automatic classification of shoe outsole designs. *Forensic Science International* 82 (1): 21–31.

Gisolf, F., Malgoezar, A., Baar, T., and Geradts, Z. (2013). Improving source camera identification using a simplified total variation based noise removal algorithm. *Digital Investigation* 10 (3): 207–214.

Grigoras, C. (2007). Applications of ENF criterion in forensic audio, video, computer and telecommunication analysis. *Forensic Science International* 167 (2): 136–145.

Grigoras, C. (2010). Statistical tools for multimedia forensics. In: *Audio Engineering Society Conference: 39th International Conference: Audio Forensics: Practices and Challenges.* Audio Engineering Society.

Hinton, G.E., Osindero, S., and Teh, Y.-W. (2006). A fast learning algorithm for deep belief nets. *Neural Computation* 18 (7): 1527–1554.

Horsman, G. (2016). Unmanned aerial vehicles: a preliminary analysis of forensic challenges. *Digital Investigation* 16: 1–11.

van Houten, W., Alberink, I., and Geradts, Z. (2011). Implementation of the likelihood ratio framework for camera identification based on sensor noise patterns. *Law, Probability and Risk* 10 (2): 149–159.

Huijbregtse, M. and Geradts, Z. (2009). Using the ENF criterion for determining the time of recording of short digital audio recordings. In: *Computational Forensics,* 116–124. Berlin, Heidelberg: Springer.

Karaküçük, A., Dirik, A.E., Sencar, H.T., and Memon, N.D. (2015). Recent advances in counter PRNU based source attribution and beyond. In: *Proceedings of SPIE – The International Society for Optical Engineering,* 9409. https://doi.org/10.1117/12.2182458.

Kloosterman, A., Mapes, A., Geradts, Z. et al. (2015). The interface between forensic science and technology: how technology could cause a paradigm shift in the role of forensic institutes in the criminal justice system. *Philosophical Transactions of the Royal Society* B370 (1674): 20140264.

Koenig, B.E. and Lacey, D.S. (2012). Forensic authenticity analyses of the header data in re-encoded WMA files from small Olympus audio recorders. *Journal of the Audio Engineering Society* 60 (4): 255–265.

Kurzweil, R. (2005). *The Singularity Is Near: When Humans Transcend Biology.* Penguin.

Lillis, David, Brett Becker, Tadhg O'Sullivan, Mark Scanlon Current Challenges and Future Research Areas for Digital Forensic Investigation. arXiv:1604.03850 (2016).

Lukas, J., Fridrich, J., and Goljan, M. (2006). Digital camera identification from sensor pattern noise. *IEEE Transactions on Information Forensics and Security* 1 (2): 205–214.

Manjunath, B.S., Salembier, P., and Sikora, T. (2002). *Introduction to MPEG-7: Multimedia Content Description Interface*, vol. 1. Wiley.

Martini, B. and Choo, K.-K.R. (2014). Cloud forensic technical challenges and solutions: a snapshot. *IEEE Cloud Computing* (4): 20–25.

Milliet, Q., Delémont, O., and Margot, P. (2014). A forensic science perspective on the role of images in crime investigation and reconstruction. *Science and Justice* 54 (6): 470–480.

Mishra, M. and Adhikary, M.C. (2013). Digital image tamper detection techniques – a comprehensive study. *International Journal of Computer Science and Business Informatics* 2 (1): 91–102.

Nikkel, B.J. (2014). Fostering incident response and digital forensics research. *Digital Investigation* 11 (4): 249–251.

Pollitt, M. and Craiger, P. (2014). Educating the next generation of cyber-forensic professionals. In: *Advances in Digital Forensics X*, 327–335. Berlin, Heidelberg: Springer.

Popejoy, A.L. (2015). Digital and multimedia forensics justified: an appraisal on professional policy and legislation. Dissertation University of Colorado Denver.

Quintana, M., Uribe, S., Sánchez, F., and Álvarez, F. (2015). Recommendation techniques in forensic data analysis: a new approach. In: *6th International Conference on Imaging for Crime Prevention and Detection (ICDP-15)*. IET.

Rahman, S. and Khan, M.N.A. (2015). Review of live forensic analysis techniques. *International Journal of Hybrid Information Technology* 8 (2): 379–388.

Sansurooah, K. and Keane, B. (2015). The spy in your pocket: smartphones and geo-location data. In: *13th Australian Digital Forensics Conference*, Western Australia, 4–18.

Scientific Working Group for Digital Evidence (2014). *SWGDE Best Practices for Handling Damaged Mobile Devices (Draft)*. SWGDE.

Siiman, L.A., Pedaste, M., Tõnisson, E. et al. (2014). A review of interventions to recruit and retain ICT students. *International Journal of Modern Education and Computer Science (IJMECS)* 6 (3): 45.

Slot, A. and Geradts, Z.J.M.H. (2014). The possibilities and limitations of forensic hand comparison. *Journal of Forensic Sciences* 59 (6): 1559–1567.

Whitcomb, C. (2002). An historical perspective of digital evidence. *International Journal of Digital Evidence* 1 (1): 8–20.

Zuech, R., Khoshgoftaar, T.M., and Wald, R. (2015). Intrusion detection and big heterogeneous data: a survey. *Journal of Big Data* 2 (1): 1–41.

CHAPTER 4

A look at the future of forensic engineering science

Thomas L. Bohan

Forensic Specialties Accreditation Board,Colorado Springs, CO, USA
American Academy of Forensic Sciences,Colorado Springs, CO, USA

"The future": a preface

Thinking about my assignment to address the future of engineering forensic science led me to reflect on what it means anyway to talk of "the future." As a boy growing up in the 1940s and 1950s, I had a keen sense of what this meant, one informed by my love of science fiction. The world of "the future" was to be one shatteringly different from my own, a world from which I could look back to my childhood and say something like "Wow, this is really different. It's *definitely* The Future." Sixty-five years later looking back, I can say:

> Wow. This really *is* different, shatteringly different from the world of my youth.

But I can also say:

> Not one of the elements now convincing me that "yes, this is *the future*" was envisioned by predictions in the press or images in my mind when I was a child.

Therefore, instead of plucking from my imagination predictions about "the future" in engineering forensic science, I am going to address what the engineering sciences *need* to do, first, regarding our flawed criminal justice system and second, regarding technology the world outside the courtroom desperately needs.

The Future of Forensic Science, First Edition. Edited by Daniel A. Martell.
© 2019 John Wiley & Sons Ltd. Published 2019 by John Wiley & Sons Ltd.

4.1 Junk law in the courtroom

The justice system's flaw is its failure to recognize its inability to resolve internally the issues of scientific validity, an inability compounded by its continued pursuit of such resolution. Some of those who ponder such things believe that behind *Daubert*,[1] the first decision regarding scientific evidence in the long history of the Supreme Court of the United States was the book that introduced "junk science" into popular usage (Huber 1991). The book was written not by a scientist, but by a lawyer who comes off as an apologist for defendants in products liability actions. Its "junk" is selective, being limited to expert testimony proffered by products-liability *plaintiffs* (Lederer and Burdick 1958).[2] Moreover, there was no reference to expert testimony in criminal trials, where the stakes are considerably higher.

Ask a scientist to identify "junk science," and you will be given examples such as cold fusion (Taubes 1993), crystal healing, *N*-rays, and perpetual motion machines. Indeed, anything introduced through a press conference or a constituent-supporting politician rather than peer-reviewed publications. Or something similar to polywater, which made it into the refereed literature but was ultimately an embarrassment to the scientists who first reported it—and more so to those who jumped on the bandwagon—when it turned out to be not replicable in anything other than capillary tubes from a particular Soviet manufacturer, which uses the term "pathological science" (National Academy of Sciences, National Academy of Engineering (US), and Institute of Medicine (US) Committee on Science, Engineering, and Public Policy 2009). These are examples of junk ("pathological") science. In contrast, placing before a jury expert testimony based on a never-validated theory is junk *law*.

First-year law school stuff: the party proffering evidence has the burden of establishing the reliability of that evidence. A judge permitting a prosecutor to place before a jury expert testimony that cannot be shown to arise from a valid theory or a technique has contaminated

---

[1] *Daubert v Merrell Dow Pharmaceuticals, Inc.*, 113 S.Ct.2786 (1993).
[2] Huber's book has been cited continually for the "junk science" phrase, though probably exclusively by those who have never read it, reminiscent of the pejorative "ugly American" used by millions unaware that it referred not to the villain but to the *hero* of the phrase-coining novel.

the courtroom with junk law.[3] Thanks primarily to forensic DNA, it has been discovered that such junk law has caused or contributed to the incarceration of hundreds of persons innocent of the heinous crimes with which they had been charged (Garrett and Neufeld 2009). Moreover, it can be inferred that thousands more have been incarcerated following convictions not testable through DNA analysis. It seems clear that these wrongful conviction revelations fueled the work producing the National Research Council Report (2009) (NAS Report) that continues to alter the forensic landscape in the United States. (Ironically, the NAS Report had a far different thrust and effect than that sought by those who lobbied Congress for it to be financed (Bohan 2010).)

The perpetuation of junk law is inherent in our adversarial system of justice and not the fault of incompetent trial judges failing at the "gatekeeper" role assigned them by *Daubert*. There is little incentive for the lawyer proffering expert testimony into evidence to exploring what underlies that testimony. Quite the opposite; when lack-of-validation objections are raised in opposition to the testimony's admission, the profferer will argue strenuously to the trial judge in favor of admission. The judge, in most cases a scientist neither by education nor inclination, will typically admit the testimony, leaving its "weight" to be assigned by a lay jury. This phenomenon explains how the cochair of the committee that prepared the NAS Report—in spite of being a federal judge with trial law experience—could have been shocked to learn of the lack of validation of traditional forensic practices.[4] Four years in preparation, the NAS Report asserted that *no* crime-lab forensic practice other than DNA identification had underlying scientific validation.

It is telling that the sole crime-lab practice found in the NAS Report to have been validated is the only one that traveled from scientific research labs to the crime labs. Only outside of the courtroom can the tests be carried out that will validate or invalidate—or most likely, define the range of validity more narrowly than has traditionally been assumed—of forensic practices and hence of the expert testimony

---

[3] The same is true of a judge permitting a defense attorney to do this. However, since the days of *Frye*, courts have been much more adept at keeping out faulty science supporting the defense.
[4] Personal comment to author from Judge Harry T. Edwards, April 2009.

based on them. This was the thrust of the 2016 report from the President's Council of Advisors on Science and Technology (PCAST),[5] which advised halting the admission into evidence of testimony based on many current forensic practices until independent scientific research into those practices could be carried out.

Alongside a group of physicians advocating evidence-based legal medicine, engineering science practitioners are testifying in defense of persons accused of infanticide based on a never-tested theory: the "shaken baby syndrome" (SBS) theory. I suggest that, if and when this theory is broadly accepted to be bogus, it will appear retrospectively that we have been in the midst of a Kuhnian (Kuhn 1962) "scientific revolution."

The SBS theory and the fact that a dispute as to its validation gained visibility with the Louise Woodward trial of 1997 (Haberman 2015). Testifying for the defense was prominent medical practitioners and researchers such as neurosurgeon Ayub Ommaya, MD, pioneering traumatic brain injury specialist and long-time neurosurgery chief for the National Institutes of Health (Holly 2008), along with biomechanical engineer Lawrence Thibault, PhD, longtime Chair of the School of Bioengineering at the University of Pennsylvania. *The Syndrome* (Goldsmith 2014), a film regarding SBS theory contains a great deal of footage from the Woodward trial, including the testimony of expert witnesses for the prosecution such as neuroradiologist, Patrick Barnes, MD, then associated with the Harvard Medical School.[6] Following the Woodward trial, reports Dr. Barnes, he read for the first time the biomechanical and other scientific literature regarding the mechanisms alleged to result in the SBS and realized that he had been incorrect in adhering to the belief he had been taught in medical school concerning it.[7] I had a similar enlightenment, in late 1998. Having been invited under the American Institute of Physics "Visiting Scientist In Physics" program to speak at Boise State University, I was asked by the head of the university's Department of Physics to review the literature on SBS and present my findings regarding

---

[5] https://obamawhitehouse.archives.gov/blog/2016/09/20/pcast-releases-report-forensic-science-criminal-courts (accessed 30 January 2017).
[6] Now Professor and Chief of Pediatric Radiology of the Stanford University Medical Center.
[7] *The Syndrome*, op cit (Personal disclosure: I appear for several seconds at one point the film).

the physical evidence supporting the theory as a part of my visit.[8] The enlightenment consisted of my discovering that there was *no* scientific support for the theory and that the totality of the literature consisted of a conjecture followed by authors quoting the conjecture and one another and their "clinical experience." Nevertheless, since 1995, SBS theory has been implemental in convicting and sentencing hundreds of people with no prior criminal records to long prison terms and even death (Hoffberger 2016). Throughout this period, engineering science practitioners have joined with pathologists and other physicians knowledgeable in the basic application of Newton's laws, to write and to testify the lack of scientific basis for concluding that the SBS theory is correct. More importantly, in light of the need to address scientific matters outside the fog of the adversarial system, they have measured the forces exerted on newborn-infant models by shaking and dropping.

The SBS theory is unique within criminology in that it both asserts that a crime has been committed *and* identifies the criminal. Presented with a dead infant exhibiting retinal hemorrhages, a subdural hematoma, and cerebral swelling (the "triad" (Tuerkheimer 2014)), the theory's adherents assert that the child was murdered by the last person holding the conscious child, specifically that person shook the baby to death. Characteristic of this theory is its application when there are no other injuries—most notably *no neck injuries*—displayed by the supposed victim. Indeed, cases exist where two of the three "triad" elements are missing, and the caretaker was tried for murder and based on nothing more than retinal hemorrhages in the decedent.

In 2004, the Engineering Sciences Section cosponsored an AAFS workshop on the SBS theory and biomechanics of head trauma (Lantz and Bohan 2004). By that year, a clear professional delineation had developed between SBS theory supporters and those asserting that it had no scientific basis. The former group was made up entirely of physicians, to the exclusion of engineers and physical scientists, and this continues to be the case. In contrast, the latter group is made

---

[8] Personal communication from Richard Reimann, PhD, currently a member of the Engineering Sciences Section of the AAFS. This led to my presentation *Shaken Baby Syndrome: A Critical Review of the Literature*, delivered at Boise State University, December 1998.

up of physicians advocating for evidence-based medicine[9] along with engineers and physical scientists, including a number of Engineering Science Section Members and Fellows. See, for example, the recent summary work of Lee and Lloyd (2016; see also, cited therein, Lloyd et al. 2011).

It has become clear through court cases and professional literature of the past 10 years that adherents of the SBS theory and those in opposition are talking past one another. No argument, whether based on Newton's laws *or on experiment*, has been able to sway any member of the former group, the attitude of which is reflected by sworn testimony such as the following:

> ...the whole point of biomechanic studies is to create what we know happens ....biomechanic models have yet to recreate what happens in nature...once those biomechanic models create what we know happens, they will be very valuable for us ...[10] (Emphasis added)

Although such an attitude is the antithesis of a scientific approach regardless of the question, it is probably no more than the stubbornness of the scientists who adhere to an "old paradigm" in Kuhn's model of how scientific change comes about. Of course, the personal consequences to others of this SBS paradigm adherence are much more serious. Kuhn saw only two sides to a scientific revolution,[11] whereas the SBS theory revolution—when testimony based on SBS joins that based on "bullet lead analysis," (National Research Council 2004) "voice prints," (National Research Council 1979), and "trial by ordeal,"(Bohan 2009) as barred from the courtroom—will take place in a four-sided arena.

---

[9] Among them are hundreds of medical practitioners in this country and abroad, including several Fellows of the Pathology/Biology Section of the AAFS. Many of them appear in a 2015 documentary. (Goldsmith op cit. Personal disclosure: I appear for several seconds at one point the film.)

[10] Jill Glick, MD, Professor of Pediatrics, University of Chicago testifying for the prosecution in the first-degree murder trial *Fleming v Reiken*, 19 February 2009, Iroquois County, Illinois, Cir. Ct.

[11] In the world of Kuhn, even as a new paradigm (at root a scientific theory) better explaining experimental observations than the one replaced, scientists who came of professional age under the old paradigm continue to cling to it. Kuhn's contribution to the philosophy of science was to point out the difficulty of convincing this group (side) to change its beliefs, even in the face of physical evidence. The other "side" comprises those who have adopted the new paradigm.

Kuhn's 1962 thesis, which came to dominate thinking in the philosophy of science within two years of its emergence (and along the way boosted the word "paradigm" and the phrase "paradigm shift" into essentially every corner of the English language), accomplished this by turning upside down the popular idea of how science is done, which accomplishment included emphasizing the difficulty of getting a theory's adherents to abandon it once it has been displaced. The first published link between Kuhn's *Structure of Scientific Revolutions*[12] was by Tuerkheimer (2009, 2014).

4.2 Forensic engineering sciences and needs of the modern world at large

Engineering science[13] practitioners include rocket scientists, physicists, medical-device designers, traffic engineers, chemists, developers, and testers of materials, fire investigators, environmental engineers—indeed, nearly every engineering specialty and all categories of physical science. As such, they were involved in the three-way dance carried out by product designer manufacturers, the public, and the legal system throughout the twentieth century, a dance that shaped the objects small and grand that define our society. In some quarters, it was referred to as tombstone technology. Mass production released products to a public numbering in the tens of millions whose use of them revealed injury- and death-causing defects not otherwise obvious. A feedback loop enlisting forensic scientists and the legal system then caused the products to be redesigned so as to minimize or eliminate those defects. It was really an iterative process, as the new designs would themselves have defects, but over 100+ years of operation, the process resulted in immense safety improvements. Moving into and through the twenty-first century, this dance will continue, but with a qualitative change arising from the electronic monitoring and control that has entered our world. The public is well aware of some of the monitoring—and

---

[12] Kuhn, op cit.

[13] Forensic engineering science is a term of art within the AAFS, being defined to include all of the traditional engineering fields plus the physical sciences as applied to forensic practice.

resents to varying degree: government surveillance; "black boxes"[14] in motor vehicles; websites that surreptitiously collect user data. But it already goes far beyond that, most importantly in terms of control: microprocessor systems track and control our airplanes, automobiles (e.g., power distribution to the respective wheels to enhance directional stability), ventilation systems, surgical procedures, communication, cameras, etc. Reportedly, but not surprisingly, such systems are now available for such individualized activities as ocean surfing and those even more personal (Silverman 2016). Microprocessor-linked controls are data-based, they *produce* data, and they occasionally malfunction. Planes crash, surgical suites catch on fire, and software-based building and highway designs incorporate flaws that injure and kill. Because of the modern role of electronic monitoring and control of product design and operation, the resolution of future civil disputes arising from these failures will require practitioners from the forensic engineering sciences to an even greater extent than they did during last century's product-liability litigation.

Another wholly modern realm of forensic technology comprises the fight against terrorism,[15] sometimes characterized as the effort to provide security to persons in public places. Although still a small part of forensic engineering science, it is a part through which its practitioners may be making their most important contributions to world societies in the years to come. It is necessary only to cite a few examples.

Although there is reason to doubt how much the cause of inflight security has been advanced by the multiple intrusions, we currently accept as a condition of boarding flights, there is no question how much engineering science went into such components of that intrusion as the "phone booths" that, as first designed, produced—one

---

[14] All automobiles produced since the late 1990s incorporate "crash data recorders" in which information about the automobile's speed, etc., during a period of time prior to a crash are stored for subsequent retrieval. The "black box" designation is carried over from the informal name assigned to flight data recorders in airplanes.

[15] Terrorism in the form of indiscriminate killing of tens of persons goes all the way back to the first public availability of dynamite in the nineteenth century. However, because such events were rare and isolated and because modern technology provides a handful of individuals the capacity to kill thousands in a single event, what we now call terrorism is a continuing activity of recent origin.

by one—images of naked passengers holding their hands above their heads, and now, after a software revision, produce a stylized human body to address modesty concerns while conveying the same information regarding what is accompanying the scanned apart from his or her clothes. As the recent attacks at airports in Brussels and Istanbul illustrate, the whole idea of security for the flying public needs rethinking. Meanwhile, basic work in a far more important area remains to be prioritized, but presumably will be eventually. I refer to the development of means to spot such items as a "suitcase nuke" hidden among the millions of tons of cargo daily traversing the world's seaports. As early as 12 September 2001, this was recognized as a far greater threat to civil society than an airborne passenger with a bomb, and yet a threat that has not yet been addressed. Monitoring cargo ships for radiation when the radiation of importance is the low-level alpha radiation from plutonium is not the solution. Yet, to all appearances, this is the only approach implemented till date, re the continuing weakness of the nation's defenses against terror delivered by cargo ship (Brill 2016). And then, there are billions of pieces of mail daily passing through the nation's post offices and into its neighborhoods and centers of commerce. What is needed from the engineering sciences is a nonintrusive, nondelaying means to probe those pieces of mail for biological weapons and for evidence that suspected terrorists are using the mails. Given the efficiency of electronic-communication surveillance (carried out with the assistance of the forensic engineering sciences), terrorist attacks may now be more securely generated and coordinated through the international postal services than through the Internet. One might expect, therefore, that some forensic engineering scientists are currently trying to develop a way to rapidly scan envelopes for traces of DNA characteristic of suspected terrorists.

With would-be terrorists less sanguine about explicit exchanges on "social media" than before, a group of forensic physicists at the University of Miami report that through "mining" ISIS-friendly websites for more subtle indicators, they are developing early-alert algorithms to enable Internet-based warnings of impending attacks (Johnson et al. 2016; also see Belluck 2016).

Acknowledgments

The author is pleased to acknowledge the suggestions and other assistance provided by AAFS Fellows Adam Aleksander, PhD, Peter Alexander, PhD, James Hyzer, PhD, David Pienkowski, PhD, and Walter Goldstein, PhD, PE from the Engineering Sciences Section, and John Plunkett, MD and Jan Leestma, MD from the Pathology/Biology Section.

References

Belluck, P. (2016). Fighting ISIS with an Algorithm, Physicists try to Predict Attacks. *The New York Times* (16 June)

Bohan, T.L. (2009). *Crashes and Collapses*. Facts on File, 313 pp + xxi, at 16.

Bohan, T.L. (2010). Review of strengthening forensic science in the United States: a path forward. *Journal of Forensic Sciences* 55: 560–564.

Brill, S. (2016). Is America safer? *The Atlantic Monthly* (September).

Garrett, B.L. and Neufeld, P.J. (2009). Invalid forensic science testimony and wrongful convictions. *Virginia Law Review* 95: 1–97, at 15.

Goldsmith, M. (2014). *The Syndrome*. Los Angeles: ReSet Films.

Haberman, C. (2015). Shaken baby syndrome: a diagnosis that divides the medical world. *The New York Times* (13 September).

Hoffberger, C. (2016). Death watch: shaken science. *The Austin Chronicle* (17 June), 35 (42).

Holly, J. (2008). Ayub K. Ommaya, 78; neurosurgeon and authority on brain injuries. *Washington Post* (14 July).

Huber, P.W. (1991). *Galileo's Revenge: Junk Science in the Courtroom*. Basic Books.

Johnson, N.F., Zheng, M., Vorobyeva, Y. et al. (2016). New online ecology of adversarial aggregates: ISIS and beyond. *Science* 352: 1459–1463.

Kuhn, T.S. (1962). *The Structure of Scientific Revolutions*. Chicago: University of Chicago Press.

Lederer, W. and Burdick, E. (1958). *The Ugly American*. New York: W.W. Norton.

Lee, W.E. III and Lloyd, J.D. (2016). Biomechanical, epidemiologic, and forensic considerations of pediatric head injuries. In: *Forensic Epidemiology* (ed. M. Freeman and M. Zeegers), 231–259. Academic Press.

Lloyd, J.D., Willey, E.N., Galaznik, J.G. et al. (2011). Biomechanical evaluation of head kinematics during infant shaking versus pediatric activities of daily living. *Journal of Forensic Biomechanics* 2: 1–9.

National Academy of Sciences, National Academy of Engineering (US) and Institute of Medicine (US) Committee on Science, Engineering, and Public Policy (2009). *On Being a Scientist: A Guide to Responsible Conduct in Research*, 3e. Washington, DC: National Academies Press.

National Research Council (1979). *On the Theory and Practice of Voice Identification*. Washington, DC, 174p.: The National Academies Press.

National Research Council (2004). *Forensic Analysis: Weighing Bullet Lead Evidence*. Washington, DC: National Academy Press.

National Research Council (2009). *Strengthening Forensic Science in the United States: A Path Forward*. Washington, DC, 328 pages plus xx: The National Academies Press.

Silverman, J. (2016). All knowing. *The New York Times Magazine* (19 June).

Taubes, G. (1993). *Bad Science: The Short Life and Weird Times of Cold Fusion*. New York: Random House.

Tuerkheimer, D. (2009). Science-dependent prosecution and the problem of epistemic contingency: a study of shaken baby syndrome. *Alabama Law Review* 62 (3): 513–569, at 558.

Tuerkheimer, D. (2014). *Flawed Convictions: "Shaken Baby Syndrome" and the Inertia of Injustice*. New York: Oxford University Press.

Patrick E. Lantz and Thomas L. Bohan. 2004. Forensic science, evidence based medicine, and the "Shaken Baby Syndrome". *Proceedings, American Academy of Forensic Sciences*, Annual Meeting, Dallas, Texas (16–21 February). p. 12, AAFS, Colorado Springs, CO.

CHAPTER 5

General section history: look at two disciplines and a review of standards, certifications, and education

John E. Gerns

American Academy of Forensic Sciences, Colorado Springs, CO, USA

5.1 Introduction

The future of the forensic sciences, including the various disciplines represented in the General Section, will have developed standards to ensure that their techniques are scientifically valid and able to withstand challenges in the judicial system. This chapter will concentrate on two subsections of the General Section in order to emphasize the magnitude of their respective discipline. Those subsections will be Medicolegal Death Investigators and Forensic Veterinarians. In addition, a brief history of government entity's review of the forensic sciences will be explored along with their impact on the forensic sciences; particularly, Medicolegal Death Investigators.

The General Section of the American Academy of Forensic Science is the most diverse discipline within the Academy. From Accounting to Veterinarian Medicine, it provides a broad spectrum of 15 forensic science specialties, all of which assist in resolving questions associated with investigations or litigations. Since its inception in 1968, the General Section has provided an avenue for new evolving disciplines to be part of the Academy and share their knowledge, experience, and application of techniques to the membership and the forensic science world.

The Future of Forensic Science, First Edition. Edited by Daniel A. Martell.

The General Forensic Section members believe we are the present and future of the Academy. We have moved from "At Large' members in 1953 to the "Gate Keepers" of the American Academy of Forensic Sciences (AAFS) today. It is through our section that forensic expertise is first identified, vetted, and accepted after a critical review of the forensic specialties to protect the integrity of the Academy. The ultimate goal of these new experts is to become a separate section. The Academy acknowledged in 1990 that the General Section was the "Mother of the Academy" because our section members took their responsibilities as a serious trust in establishing new forensic disciplines. This process has been repeated several times with the first being Forensic Anthropology in 1973 and the latest, Digital and Multimedia Sciences in 2008. Our latest accepted discipline is Forensic Veterinary Sciences, concerned with the health and welfare of animals through the recovery, identification, and examination of material evidence of inhumane destruction, treatment, abuse, neglect, or illicit trade in animals or animal parts for illegal purposes. Veterinary technologists and technicians perform medical tests under the supervision of a licensed veterinarian to treat or to help veterinarians diagnose the illnesses and injuries of animals (Dr. G. Pusillo, Forensic Veterinary Science, Briefing and Personal Communication).

5.2 Forensic veterinary science

Normally, when we think of a veterinarian, we envision an individual who is primarily involved in assessing an animal's ailments, then rendering medical assistance to that animal. Just like a physician examining a child's injuries, sometimes the cause can be attributed to maltreatment. The physician is then required to report the suspected abuse to the proper authorities for investigation to safeguard the child. Veterinarians have the same mandated reporting requirements for abuse. According to the chart provided by the American Veterinary Medical Association (AVMA) on 1 October 2010, only 14 states have mandated reporting for veterinarians of suspected cruelty to animals or animal fighting, and six states allow the reporting (Arkow et al. 2011). In the world of veterinarian science, a new discipline of Veterinary Forensics conducts investigations to determine the cause of the ailment, injury, or death. But this discipline has a broad array of multidisciplinary areas of animal expertise: nutrition, medicine, production, genetics, behavior, pathology, physiology, husbandry, biochemistry, and welfare. As Dr. Pusillo states, "Forensic Veterinary science must be inclusive of professionals that are experts in their respective fields." To illustrate the scope of these disciplines, we will look at Commercial Animal Production. This category includes numerous subcategories of why the animals are raised: human consumption; production of wool, hair, fur, skin, and antlers; performance activity; providing replacements and breeding stock; zoological collections; experimental subjects; urine and blood for research and composition of vaccines and medications; pet industry; and service animals. Proper investigations into allegations of abuse in any of these production categories require individuals trained and experienced in each type of production situation. One area of Forensic Veterinary Science that gets much media exposure is animal cruelty. This can include investigations of cruelty to domestic pets, production of livestock such as cattle and sheep, and also horses to name a few. The key to successful investigations into cruelty is education, experience, and training in the respective field. For example Dr. Pusillo illustrates how a very well cared for draft horse could be viewed as cruel and mistreated in the eyes of a veterinarian who specializes in small domestic animals. Investigating allegations of horse maltreatment requires additional expertise than your normal licensed veterinarian. According to Dr. Pusillo, they should have a BS, MS, and PhD in animal husbandry, production, nutrition, and physiology along with a minimum of 10 years of experience in these fields. Plus, he believes they should have a demonstrated ability to write scientific papers and interpret published data. And five years of expert witness experience and investigative knowledge put into practice within the legal system. To emphasize who would typically request someone with expertise in veterinary horse forensics, the following is a sampling of investigations requiring that expertise: (i) law enforcement agencies investigating potential horse cruelty incidents; (ii) insurance companies investigating a suspicious death of a highly insured horse; (iii) feed companies accused of providing improper horse nutrition products to customers claiming a specific product caused horse abnormalities, decrease in performance, or death; (iv) insurance companies that insure these feed companies; and (v) horse racetrack officials investigating illegal substances found in preracing or postracing tests.

The final discipline that will be described within Veterinary Forensics is a nutritionist. Although they are not currently represented in AAFS, they play a key role in animal welfare. According to Dr. Pusillo, animal nutrition is the most important category of commercial animal health, production, and welfare since animals have to eat and drink every day. Forensic nutritionists determine not only what might be affecting a group of animals but also the impact a food imbalance, contaminant, or additive has on the final product. They are involved in investigating death of large numbers of production animals; determining which nutritional inputs might have a harmful effect on humans consuming animal-based products; supporting local law enforcement agencies to see if animal foods are poisoned or contaminated by deliberate actions; investigating what nutrient supplements are used illegally or that are in noncompliance with regulatory agencies; and help determine if animals were fed tainted feeds in order to collect insurance money associated with performance activities or breeding value. A typical day for a forensic animal nutritionist can include the following: recreate a ration for a specific species that is part of an investigation. This involves using advanced nutrition knowledge and complex computer programs; check feed samples under a microscope; photograph feed samples as presented and under microscopic conditions; conduct feeding trials of retained samples and feeds under investigation; analyze feed samples for expected nutrients; analyze feed samples for adulterants, insects, mold, mycotoxins, or other potential contaminants; inspect feeding equipment to see if appropriate for species and production expectations; inspect storage facilities and structures intended to keep feed safe and wholesome; inspect and test mixing and distribution systems of feed to be sure if they meet minimum standards for the species and production levels expected; review and document all environmental conditions that have an influence on the daily ration fed; and test water sources.

As you can see, the discipline of Forensic Veterinary Science is very complex and dynamic. As in any investigation, it requires a multidisciplinary approach to successfully resolve an allegation of cruelty or nutritional irregularities. Similar to many of the forensic science disciplines, they take their job very seriously and strive for truth and justice. The Veterinarian's Oath describes that dedication, "Veterinarian's Oath (USA) Being admitted to the profession of veterinary medicine, I solemnly swear to use my scientific knowledge and skills for the benefit of society through the protection of animal health and welfare, the prevention and relief of animal suffering, the conservation of animal resources, the promotion of public health, and the advancement of medical knowledge. I will practice my profession conscientiously, with dignity, and in keeping with the principles of veterinary medical ethics. I accept as a lifelong obligation the continual improvement of my professional knowledge and competence." There are over 40 disciplines in AVMA ranging from Academics to Zoological Medicine (Arkow et al. 2011); AVMA Policies (www.avma .org/kb/policies/pages/default.aspx).

The AVMA has over 200 policies ranging from abuse and neglect of animals to zoonotic infections. Policies are the guiding principles of the association. These policies fall into three categories. AVMA professional policies provide guidance on the practice of veterinary medicine. Endorsed policies are policies adopted by other groups and supported by the AVMA. Administrative policies are primarily internal and direct the operation of the Association.

The AVMA encourages its members to voluntarily adhere to policies impacting the practice of veterinary medicine, as these policies are developed by peers on behalf of the profession. AVMA policies are not, and do not supersede, law or regulation. The AVMA Principles of Veterinary Medical Ethics are unique in that violation of these may result in disciplinary action by the AVMA.

Many forensic science disciplines have created an association designed to afford its members the opportunity to share their knowledge, receive new training, and develop networks to assist them in their professional and investigative development. The current association for forensic veterinarians is the International Veterinary Forensic Sciences Association (IVFSA).

In May 2008, the American Society for the Prevention of Cruelty to Animals (ASPCA) and the Maples Center for Forensic Medicine at the University of Florida College of Medicine partnered to host a conference on veterinary forensic sciences. This conference was organized by the ASPCA's Dr. Randall Lockwood and Dr. Melinda Merck, and Dr. Jason Byrd with the University of Florida. The majority of attendees at the Veterinary Forensic Sciences Conference voted to create the IVFSA, and additionally voted to make Veterinary Forensic Sciences Conference an annual event.

The purpose of the IVFSA is to (i) promote the health, welfare, and safety of animals through the fostering of current and novel techniques of forensic science and crime scene processing to circumstances of animal abuse, neglect, cruelty, fighting, and death; (ii) apply forensic science techniques to legal investigations involving animals as the victim of criminal offenses and civil disputes; (iii) educate the animal welfare community, law enforcement, crime scene analysts, forensic scientists, veterinarians, attorneys, judges, and pathologists on the application of forensic science techniques and crime scene processing methods to cases of animal abuse, neglect, cruelty, fighting, and death; (iv) inform the law enforcement and legal community on the various scientific disciplines that can be utilized for the interpretation of collected physical evidence related to any crime scene where an animal's presence or absence is relevant; and (v) advance and foster excellence in the veterinary forensic sciences (www.ivfsa.org/about).

5.3 Certification: introduction

Regardless of the investigative technique, it is critical that an established and accepted procedure, once adopted by the respective scientific community, is adhered to when used. Training on new techniques must be developed to ensure their application is accomplished through established standards. Certifying organizations ensure these approved standards are incorporated into a process. Certification promotes standardization.

5.4 Certification—ABMDI

In order to put the importance of certifications in perspective, the development of the American Board of Medicolegal Death Investigators (ABMDI) is described. ABMDI details its evolution along with the various government entities and policies that not only sustained its existence but also availed funds to assist in its certification program.

The National Research Council's report (National Academy of Sciences 2009) stated that no person (public or private) shall be allowed to practice in a forensic science discipline or testify as a forensic science professional without relevant certification. Certification provides general confidence by promoting standardization and recognizing individuals who demonstrate proficiency in the standards and practice necessary to properly perform job duties (Howe 2011).

Currently, there is only one widely recognized and accredited certifying body for medicolegal death investigators, the ABMDI. The ABMDI was established in 1998 as a not-for-profit, independent professional certification board to promote the highest standards of practice for medicolegal death investigators. In 2005, the ABMDI was first accredited by the Forensic Specialties Accreditation Board (FSAB) and reaccredited in 2010 and 2015. The goal of FSAB is to establish a mechanism whereby the forensic community can assess, recognize, and monitor organizations or professional boards that certify individual forensic scientists or other forensic specialists.

Although the certification process for medicolegal death investigators has been established, there still remain obstacles for medicolegal death investigators to become certified. Funding of the application, examination, case load, and maintenance of certification, creates barriers, especially in smaller jurisdictions where the cost typically falls to the individual.

The National Commission on Forensic Science (NCFS) was created in 2013 as a Federal Advisory Committee to the Department of Justice (DOJ) and was like no other existing entity. The purpose of the NCFS was to represent the broadest range of interests involved, affected by, or able to improve forensic evidence. The NCFS provided recommendations to the Attorney General for forensic policy considerations (https://www.justice.gov/archives/ncfs/page/file/959356/download). The NCFS recommended in January 2015 that the Office of Justice Programs establishes a priority to use grant funds to defray the cost of ensuring that medicolegal death investigation personnel become and maintain certification, specifically by the ABMDI, by the end of 2020 (https://www.justice.gov/archives/ncfs/page/file/788026/download). There are currently 1736 Registered ABMDI Certificants and 225 Fellows, emphasizing that the recommendation is far from being realized.

ABMDI certifies individuals who have the proven knowledge and skills necessary to perform medicolegal death investigations as set forth in the National Institutes of Justice 1999 publication *Death Investigation: A Guide for the Scene Investigator* (2011 updated version available).

Since the early 1990s, forensic subject-matter experts have collaborated to improve discipline practices and build consensus standards through Scientific Working Groups (SWGs). The SWG Medicolegal Death Investigations (SWGMDI) was created in March 2011 and operated until its completion in 2014 with support from the National Institute of Justice (NIJ) through an interagency agreement with the FBI. Members were from local, state, or federal agencies, research institutions, or organizations that support medicolegal death investigations and represent the medical examiner, coroner, medicolegal death investigator, and forensic community at large.

In 2014, SWGMDI transitioned into the Organization of Scientific Area Committees (OSAC) for Forensic Science that is part of an initiative by National Institute of Standards and Technology (NIST) and the Department of Justice to strengthen forensic science in the United States.

5.5   Standards evolution—OSAC

The mission of the OSAC for Forensic Science is to strengthen the nation's use of forensic science by facilitating the development of scientifically sound forensic science standards and by promoting the adoption of those standards by the forensic science community (OSAC, Charter and Bylaws). OSAC is administered by the NIST, but the great majority of its more than 550 members are from other government agencies, academic institutions, and the private sector. These members have expertise in 25 specific forensic disciplines, as well as general expertise in scientific research, measurement science, statistics, law, and policy.

Five Scientific Area Committees (SACs) cover broadly defined forensic science topic areas and oversee 25 discipline-specific subcommittees. The subcommittees work to identify existing high-quality standards and to facilitate the development of new standards by Standards Development Organizations. Those standards, whether new or existing, can then be moved through OSAC's standards approval process. The SACs approve standards identified by the sub-committees and provide coordination when standards span multiple disciplines. After a SAC approves a standard, it forwards that standard to the Forensic Science Standards Board (FSSB) for final approval (OSAC, Terms of Reference).

The FSSB oversees the SACs and subcommittees, establishes governance rules and policies to ensure the development of quality standards, and encourages their use in the provision of forensic science services. The FSSB administers overall operation of the organization, approves standards for inclusion on the OSAC Registry, and updates and disseminates the list of approved documents. The FSSB also approves membership nominations, resolves disputes and appeals, and engages in international efforts related to forensic science standards (OSAC, FSSB Terms of Reference).

5.6 Standard evolution—ASB

The AAFS Standards Board (ASB) is an ANSI-accredited Standards Developing Organization with the purpose of providing accessible, high-quality science-based consensus forensic standards. The ASB is a wholly owned subsidiary of the AAFS, established in 2015, and accredited by the American National Standards Institute (ANSI) in 2016. The ASB is partially funded by a grant through the Laura and John Arnold Foundation.

The ASB consists of Consensus Bodies (CBs), which are open to all materially interested and affected individuals, companies, and organizations, a board of directors, and staff.

ANSI facilitates the development of American National Standards (ANS) by accrediting the procedures of standards developing organizations (SDOs). These groups work cooperatively to develop voluntary national consensus standards. Accreditation by ANSI signifies that the procedures used by the standards body in connection with the development of ANS meet the Institute's essential requirements for openness, balance, consensus, and due process.

With the approval of the National Technology Transfer and Advancement Act (NTTAA) of 1995 (Public Law 104-113), federal agencies are encouraged to utilize voluntary consensus standards wherever feasible and to participate as appropriate in voluntary consensus standards development activities. Standards that are approved as ANS satisfy all the requirements of the NTTAA.

In order to maintain ANSI accreditation, standard's developers are required to consistently adhere to a set of requirements or procedures that govern the consensus development process. These requirements are set forth in a document known as the ANSI Essential Requirements: Due process requirements for ANS (www.ansi.org/essentialrequirements).

Due process is the key to ensuring that ANSs are developed in an environment that is equitable, accessible, and responsive to the requirements of various stakeholders. The open and fair ANS process ensures that all interested and affected parties have an opportunity to participate in a standard's development. It also serves and protects the public interest since standard's developers accredited by ANSI must meet the Institute's essential requirements and other due process safeguards (ASB Guide 001, Updated, March 2018).

5.7   Education accreditation

Every journey starts with a first step. Someone interested in pursuing a career in the forensic sciences, regardless of the discipline, should start first with their collegiate education. This will set the foundation for beginning a career and will enable a successful pursuit of their forensic science goal. However, ensuring you receive the best educational foundation possible is critical to what school you select.

The mission of the Forensic Science Education Programs Accreditation Commission (FEPAC) is to maintain and to enhance the quality of forensic science education through a formal evaluation and recognition of college-level academic programs. The primary function of the commission is to develop and to maintain standards and to administer an accreditation program that recognizes and distinguishes high-quality undergraduate and graduate forensic science programs. There are currently 35 forensic science educational programs accredited.

FEPAC's conceptual development began in 1999 when an article was published in NIJ (U.S. Department of Justice 1999). In its executive summary, it emphasized that the training needs of the forensic community are immense. It addressed the educational needs of not only newcomers to the forensic science arena but also seasoned forensic science practitioners. Whether they worked in a laboratory conducting analysis or were working in the field at crime scenes, they emphasized that "Forensic scientists must stay up-to-date as new technology, equipment, methods, and techniques are developed." NIJ furthered their efforts to enhance the evolution of forensic science training needs when they created the Technical Working Group for Education and Training in Forensic Sciences (TWGED) in 2001. As a result of their research on the necessity of education and training in the forensic sciences, AAFS established an ad hoc committee called Forensic Education Program Accreditation Committee to look at how to best develop an accreditation program. In 2004, FEPAC became an official standing committee with AAFS and awarded its first accreditation in February 2004 (AAFS FEPAC Accreditation Standards, 16 May 2003, revised 12 February 2017).

5.8 Summary

The General Section of the AAFS covers a wide array of forensic science disciplines. Two disciplines, Forensic Veterinarians and Medicolegal Death Investigators were highlighted to emphasize the forensic science diversity of the section. Using ABMDI as an example of a certifying body, it detailed the evolution which led to its current state. That evolution included how varying government and organizational entities aided in its development. Forensic veterinarians illustrated the complexity of a new discipline and how it can apply to a wide range of investigations. As technology advances and new methods are developed to identify, collect, preserve, and analyze evidence, it is imperative that a structured avenue is developed to ensure investigative techniques are properly administered. A strong educational foundation should begin the journey. FEPAC continuously evaluates and identifies undergraduate and graduate schools that excel in their forensic science education. Government entities and professional organizations not only conduct research and develop policies and standards to ensure proper application and consistency, but they also assist in the procurement of funds to enable forensic science professionals to receive the proper training to achieve certification in their respective fields and develop and maintain their expertise.

Acknowledgements

Julie Howe and Dr. Gay Pusillo greatly contributed to this chapter. Their dedication to their respective forensic science disciplines along with their professionalism truly enhances the investigative missions they promote. The author is extremely grateful for their assistance and insight.

References

Arkow, P., Boyden, P., and Patterson-Kane, E. (2011). *Practical Guidance for the Effective Response by Veterinarians to Suspected Animal Cruelty, Abuse and Neglect.* AVMA.

Howe, J. (2011). Professional certification for medicolegal death investigators – ABMDI. *Academic Forensic Pathology* 1 (4): 348–355.

National Academy of Sciences 2009. Strengthening Forensic Science in the United States: A Path Forward. http://www.nap.edu/catalog/12589.html.

OSAC. Charter and Bylaws. Date of issue: 4 April (2018). /Version 1.4/Issuing Authority: Forensic Science Standards Board.

OSAC. Terms of Reference. Date of issue: 6 December 2017/Version 1.5/Issuing Authority: Forensic Science Standards Board.

OSAC. FSSB Terms of Reference. Date of issue: 6 December 2017/Version 1.6/Issuing Authority: Forensic Science Standards Board.

ASB Manual for Standards, Best Practice Recommendations, and Technical Reports, Updated, 2018.

ASB Guide 001, Updated, March 2018.

U.S. Department of Justice (Febraury 1999). Forensic Science: Review of Status and Needs. Office of Justice Programs, NCJ 173412.

CHAPTER 6

The future of forensic science: hot leads in contemporary forensic research: Jurisprudence

Carol Henderson

Consultant in Law and Forensic Science, Past President AAFS, St Petersburg Beach, FL

The relationship between the law and science and lawyers and scientists has been described as both an essential reliance and a reluctant embrace

Source: *Jasanoff 1995, pp. 204–206*

Jurisprudence has been an integral part of the American Academy of Forensic Sciences (AAFS) since its inception during the First American Medicolegal Congress in 1948. Dr. Rutherford B.H. Gradwohl, Dr. Sidney Kaye, and Mr. Orville Richardson, a then prominent St. Louis attorney, became the founders of AAFS, which is an internationally recognized academy focused on improving the justice system by promoting more reliable scientific evidence. In addition, the AAFS Jurisprudence Section stands among the first seven sections of the Academy, along with forensic pathology, forensic psychiatry, forensic toxicology, forensic immunology, police science, and questioned documents sections. Mr. Richardson's contributions, including his service as the principal author of the AAFS Constitution, legal counsel to the AAFS Administration and Secretary of the Jurisprudence Section in 1952, ensured the Academy's prospects as the largest and most effective academy of forensic sciences. In addition, Since Mr. Fred Inbau, whom served as Jurisprudence Section President

The Future of Forensic Science, First Edition. Edited by Daniel A. Martell.
© 2019 John Wiley & Sons Ltd. Published 2019 by John Wiley & Sons Ltd.

from 1955 to 1956, there have been a total of 10 Jurisprudence Section Presidents.[1]

Since its first meeting in Chicago, in 1957, the Jurisprudence Section has focused on interdisciplinary communication and education between the forensic science and legal communities. There has always been a need for reliable forensic evidence and informed lawyers and judges. Through annual meetings, scientific sessions, and publications, the Jurisprudence Section continues to ensure that scientists and lawyers alike are trained and prepared for issues that arise with forensic science.

Paralleling the original aspirations of the Academy, the Jurisprudence Section and its members have inspired confidence and respect for the forensic sciences while also strengthening the reliability and accuracy of forensic evidence. Section members have served on the National Commission on Forensic Science (NCFS)[2] in addition to serving as members on both the Legal Resource Committee (LRC) of National Institute of Standards and Technology (NIST's) Organization of Scientific Area Committees (OSAC)[3] and various subcommittees. Jurisprudence members continue to positively influence the forensic sciences while also educating scientists and attorneys who rely on the Academy's information and principles.

The Jurisprudence Section, while at 202 members, yields much influence in the forensic sciences. Judge Pamela A. W. King, JD is the Jurisprudence Section Chair for 2018–2019. She served on the NCFS. Members of the Section, including other prominent judges, practitioners, and academicians have provided numerous training sessions and

---

[1] Including Oliver Schroeder from 1963 to 1964, Jack L. Sachs, LLB, from 1966 to 1967, Edwin C. Conrad, JD, MS, from 1970 to 1971, Robert J. Joling, LLB, from 1975 to 1976, Don Harper Mills, MD, JD, from 1986 to 1987, Haskell M. Pitluck, JD, from 1995 to 1996, Kenneth E. Melson, JD, from 2003 to 2004, Carol E. Henderson, JD, from 2008 to 2009, and Betty Layne DesPortes, JD, from 2017 to 2018.

[2] The section of this chapter titled "NCFS" is based primarily on the NCFS public website and links therein, located at: Homepage: https://www.justice.gov/ncfs.

[3] The section of this chapter titled "OSAC" is based primarily on NIST's OSAC public website and links therein, located at:
Homepage: https://www.nist.gov/forensics/osac/index.cfm.
http://www.nist.gov/topics/forensic-science/organization-scientific-area-committees-osac/osac-registry/osac-approval

moot court exercises at AAFS meetings. The Jurisprudence Section continues to train members of the scientific and legal community in collaboration with many other organizations. Jurisprudence members assist AAFS[4] in its role as an American National Standards Institute (ANSI)-accredited Standards Developing Organization (SDO).[5]

The Harold A. Feder award recognizes Jurisprudence Section members who have outstanding achievements and contributions in time, service, and dedication to the Academy and the Jurisprudence Section. The award has been presented to 25 AAFS Jurisprudence Section members since the award was first presented in 1981 to Edwin Conrad, Robert J. Joling, JD, and Jack L. Sachs, JD.[6] The Jurisprudence Section continues to recognize the invaluable contributions the members have made to the scientific and legal communities, including ongoing efforts to educate lawyers and judges in the complexities of forensic science.

This chapter will describe the present state of the law of admissibility of scientific evidence. It will discuss the recent challenges in expert testimony admissibility, the development of policies and standards for forensic science practitioners, and the efforts being made to educate judges and lawyers in forensic science.

6.1 Daubert's history

Over 25 years ago, the US Supreme Court decided *Daubert v. Merrell Dow Pharmaceuticals, Inc.* (1993). The Court provided guidance to judges on assessing all forms of expert witness testimony for reliability

---

[4] AAFS is an SDO (professional organization providing leadership, standardized practices, and collaboration in forensic sciences) asbstandardsboard.org

[5] AAFS President's Message September 2015 (AAFS received $1.5 million to establish a SDO that is ANSI-accredited and intended to be used by organizations such as NIST's OSAC to vet the promulgated standard or policy).

[6] AAFS Jurisprudence Section Award (Harold A. Feder Award) Recipients: Richard Allen (1982), Jay Schwartz (1982), Don Harper Mills (1983), Oliver C. Schroeder, Jr. (1983), Arthur H. Schatz (1984), Edwin Marger (1988), James E. Starrs (1988), Haskell M. Pitluck (1991), Kenneth E. Melson (1993), Harold A. Feder (1996), Andre A. Moenssens (1998), Carol Henderson (1999), Gil Sapir (2000), Stephen A. Brunette (2001), Haskell M. Pitluck (2003), Cynthia L. Windsor (2004), Linda B. Kenney (2006), Robert J. Joling (2008), Danielle D. Ruttman (2012), Betty Layne DesPortes (2014), and Roderick T. Kennedy (2018).

and accuracy. The case set an important precedent, followed by all federal and most state courts in their attempt to determine the admissibility of both scientific and non-scientific expert testimonies.

Daubert, a civil case, hinged on the validity of the scientific methodology of the experts' opinions regarding the causal link between an anti-nausea drug, Bendectin, and birth defects. A key issue before the Court was whether the so-called "*Frye* test," which emerged from the US Supreme Court case *Frye v. United States* (1923) was the appropriate means for determining the admissibility of expert testimony or whether the Federal Rules of Evidence, which were enacted in 1975, superseded the "*Frye* test" (*Daubert* 1993, p. 584).[7] *Frye*, a criminal case, involved a determination about the admissibility of evidence from a blood pressure test, which for a time was used as a lie detection method. *Frye* held that scientific evidence is admissible if the technique upon which it is based is "sufficiently established to have gained general acceptance in the particular field in which it belongs" (*Frye* 1923, p. 1014). *Frye* was rarely cited for a quarter-century, but over time the "*Frye* test" became increasingly influential, and by the early 1980s it had been adopted by 29 states (Haack 2005).

The *Daubert* Court had to determine the status of *Frye* in relation to the Federal Rules of Evidence, Rule 702, which then stated: "If scientific, technical or other specialized knowledge will assist the trier of fact to understand the evidence or to determine a fact in issue, a witness qualified as an expert by knowledge skill, experience, training or education, may testify thereto in the form of an opinion or otherwise." The *Daubert* Court held the Federal Rules of Evidence, not *Frye*, provided the standard for admitting expert scientific evidence in a federal trial. The Federal Rules of Evidence assign the trial judge the task of ensuring that an expert's testimony is relevant and reliable. "Pertinent evidence based on scientifically valid principles will satisfy those demands." (*Daubert* 1993, p. 597). The *Daubert* Court supplemented the "general acceptance" standard with a more robust inquiry related to the accuracy, reliability, evaluation, and accreditation of the underlying principles and methodologies used by an expert witness.

---

[7] Federal Rules of Evidence (2011) Rule 702, as amended.

Since 1993, thousands of judges have cited the *Daubert* case in their decisions. The *"Daubert* test" has become the majority approach for state courts in the United States, with 39 states having adopted some form of the *Daubert,* test, while eight states, including the District of Colombia, retain the *Frye* test (Morgenstern 2016). Four other states, Virginia, North Dakota, Nevada, and Missouri, have retained a unique test for the admissibility and authentication of expert testimony. *Id.* North Dakota and Virginia have not adopted any form of the *Daubert* test or its progeny, rather they use a modified version of Federal Rule of Evidence 702. Virginia courts use a broader standard, admitting expert testimony if "it will assist trier of fact in understanding evidence." *Id.*

6.2   The *Daubert* test

The Supreme Court identified five factors to aid judges in making a preliminary assessment of whether the methodology or theory underlying expert witness testimony is scientifically valid and can properly be applied to the facts at issue. The factors are:

1. Whether the scientific methodology or theory can be and has been tested;
2. Whether the methodology or theory has been subjected to peer review and publication;
3. The known or potential error rate of the methodology or theory;
4. The existence and maintenance of standards controlling the operation of the methodology or theory used by the expert witness;
5. Whether it has widespread acceptance within the relevant scientific community (*Daubert* 1993, pp. 593–594).

6.3   Questions raised by *Daubert*

Shortly after the *Daubert* decision, many unresolved issues started to emerge. For example, the lower courts had to determine how judges were supposed to serve as gatekeepers of expert testimony. In short, are they supposed to perform a preliminary assessment of expert testimony or should the default setting be to admit such testimony and trust the examination/cross-examination process to vet it properly?

Furthermore, judges had to determine what was to be reviewed if they were going to serve as gatekeepers of scientific evidence and expert testimony. More specifically, were they to limit their attention to an expert's methods alone, or were the expert's conclusions part of their purview as well?

Another key issue was the relative importance of whether expert testimony is "scientific" in nature, and if so, whether different admissibility standards should be applied to "scientific" as opposed to "non-scientific" expert testimony. Chief Justice Rehnquist seemed to question whether there was a relevant distinction between "scientific" and "technical" evidence and if so, how judges would be able to draw such a distinction. The lower courts also had to ascertain whether they were required to strictly apply the *Daubert* factors when evaluating expert testimony or whether those factors were mere recommendations, to be applied in a non-exhaustive manner in any given case.

Over the years, the questions discussed above were further analyzed in two additional Supreme Court cases, *General Electric Co. v. Joiner* (1997) and *Kumho Tire Co. v. Carmichael* (1999), which along with *Daubert v. Merrell Dow Pharmaceuticals, Inc.* (1993) formed the so-called "*Daubert* trilogy". The *Kumho* case added clarity to the types of expert testimony to which the *Daubert* test was intended to apply. Specifically, *Kumho* established that the *Daubert* test was to be applied to all expert testimony, not simply to "scientific" expert testimony. Further, *Kumho* (p. 150) made it clear that the Federal Rule of Evidence 702 inquiry is a flexible one that allows the court to focus only on the pertinent factors in any given case to determine expert testimony admissibility. This analysis confirmed the *Daubert* test was not intended to represent a definitive checklist for the admissibility of scientific evidence.

6.4 The NAS report

In 2005, Congress recognized the importance of scientific evidence to the legal system and called for the creation of an independent forensic science committee at the National Academy of Sciences (NAS) to identify the needs of the forensic science community. The committee was asked to do the following: assess present and future resource needs of labs, medical examiner and coroner offices; identify potential scientific advances that will assist law enforcement in using forensic technologies; and determine how to disseminate best practices and guidelines to ensure quality and consistency in the use of technologies and techniques, among other tasks. This effort resulted in the 2009 report from the NAS' Committee on Identifying the Needs of the Forensic Science Community *Strengthening Forensic Science in the United States: A Path Forward* (NAS Report 2009).

The NAS Report discussed *Daubert* in detail, observing that its progeny has engendered confusion and controversy. Studies suggested that courts were less demanding in their application of *Daubert* in criminal trials, as opposed to civil trials. In particular, the NAS Report (p. 11) indicated that criminal prosecution and civil plaintiff evidence was generally given more leeway in regards to satisfying the *Daubert* admissibility test than was defendant evidence in similar cases. By requiring a more rigorous examination of experts' methodologies, the *Daubert* test required judges and lawyers to be more knowledgeable about science. Yet, as Justice Rehnquist noted, the 22 amicus briefs dealt with scientific matters "far afield of the expertise of judges" (*Daubert* 1993, p. 599). Without additional guidance regarding scientific methodologies and the reliability of standards therein, lawyers and judges may not be able to effectively explain the reliability, or unreliability, of scientific processes and evidence presented in court.

Since *Daubert*, there have been increasing challenges to forensic science, particularly in fields relying on comparison evidence. In February 2016, the Texas Forensic Science Commission approved a temporary prohibition on the admissibility of bite mark evidence until adequate standards and methodologies are developed to its admissibility (Herskovitz 2016; Palazzolo 2016). In 2013 the Federal Bureau of Investigation began reviewing FBI laboratory analyst testimony related to hair comparison analysis to identify erroneous convictions and ensure future forensic testing will be based on sufficiently accepted scientific standards (Reimer 2013). In April 2015, the FBI identified "twenty-six of 28 FBI agent/analysts provided either testimony with erroneous statements or submitted laboratory reports with erroneous statements" (FBI: National Press Release, 2015).

In response, many federal and state SDOs are working to improve the science behind scientific evidence while also producing educational material to assist judges and lawyers in understanding and explaining the principles used by a scientific expert.[8]

6.5 The national commission on forensic science and the organization of scientific area committees

Two government entities were established to address the NAS Report (2009) recommendations—the NCFS, whose mission was to develop policy, and the OSAC, whose mission is to develop discipline-specific practice standards and guidelines. The OSAC Forensic Resource Committee and the NCFS Training on Science and Law Subcommittee, were committed to greater interdisciplinary knowledge sharing between the legal and forensic science communities.

6.6 NCFS

The NCFS (2013–2017) was a Federal Advisory Committee for the Department of Justice that was created for the critical purpose of providing policy recommendations through a notice-and-comment process. It consisted of federal, state, and local forensic science

---

[8] *International Organization of Standards: TC 272 Forensic Sciences* (provides standardization and guidance to the forensic science across the world in the form of improved procedures and techniques for various forensic science disciplines) http://www.iso.org/iso/home/standards_development/list_of_iso_technical_committees/iso_technical_committee.htm?commid=4395817. Standards Development Organization (SDO) examples:
International Organization of Standards (ISO): *TC 272 Forensic Sciences*. ISO—TC 272 is planning a meeting in June 2016 to discuss new and existing standards and techniques in both scientific laboratories and field based practices throughout the world. http://www.iso.org/iso/home/standards_development/list_of_iso_technical_committees/iso_technical_committee.htm?commid=4395817. AAFS is an ANSI accredited SDO. In March 2016, AAFS began accepting applications for the formation of Consensus Bodies, which are expected to collaborate amongst members in their specific scientific interest group to produce standard practices and guidelines. http://asb.aafs.org/wp-content/uploads/2016/01/Webinar_Presentation_Slides.pdf.

service providers, scientists, academics, law enforcements officials, prosecutors, defense attorneys, and judges tasked to produce practical recommendations on how the forensic science community can improve to better effectuate the administration of justice by legal professionals. The NCFS members evaluated guidelines and standards identified by subject-matter experts, and formulated policy recommendations for the Attorney General. The NCFS worked toward strengthening the methodology and reliability of forensic sciences, enhancing quality assurance and quality control of forensic laboratories, and developing discipline-specific standards and protocols for evidence seizure, testing, analysis, and reporting by forensic practitioners (Butler 2014).

The NCFS held 13 meetings, during which it adopted 43 work products[9]: recommendations and views documents, regarding the accreditation, interoperability, and reliability of standards across forensic science disciplines. One recommendation directed attorneys and forensic service providers working on behalf of the Department of Justice to forego the use of the ambiguous term "reasonable scientific certainty" (NCFS 2016). As the NCFS stated, the use of the term "reasonable scientific certainty" by both legal professions and expert witnesses has obscured the scientific process behind expert testimony, rather than bringing clarity to it. NCFS (2016) *Recommendations to the Attorney General Regarding Use of the Term* "Reasonable Scientific Certainty."

In December 2015, the NCFS approved a recommendation to develop uniform standards to reduce contextual bias and other human factors that affect forensic science service providers (NCFS 2015a). In this recommendation the NCFS determined that particular phases of a forensic investigation should be insulated from bias-inducing evidence in order to produce scientifically accurate and reliable conclusions (NCFS 2015a). For example, witness statements that are necessary for the preliminary collection of evidence by a crime scene investigator could likely result in a biased conclusion if also known to the forensic analyst during the examination of such evidence, whether consciously or subconsciously. The NCFS

---

[9] National Commission on Forensic Science Work Products Adopted by the Commission: http://www.justice.gov/ncfs/work-products-adopted-commission.

(2015a) agreed that limiting an analyst's exposure to identifiable bias-inducing evidence would significantly increase the accuracy of forensic testing and the reliability of the conclusions drawn therefrom. It recommended that forensic science service providers and crime laboratories begin monitoring their forensic practitioners' exposure to evidence that could result in contextual, cognitive, or other forms of bias (NCFS 2015a). Practically this would mean dividing the phases of a criminal investigation into subparts: (i) collection of evidence, (ii) analysis of evidence, and (iii) conclusions formulated from analyzed evidence (NCFS 2015a).

In addition, the NCFS adopted a policy recommendation in April 2015 which set forth an implementation strategy for the universal accreditation of all forensic science disciplines (NCFS 2015b). This policy would strengthen the foundation of forensic testing and motivate federal and state crime laboratories to adhere to accepted scientific standards and procedures.

6.7 OSAC

The OSAC was partnered with the NCFS in 2013 to conduct a survey of forensic sciences and to produce guidelines and standards for individual forensic disciplines. Comprised of more than 500 forensic science practitioners nationwide, the OSAC harmonizes the viewpoints of local, state, and federal forensic science service providers in order to thoroughly evaluate and adopt nationally recognizable standards. In addition, the OSAC is responsible for identifying, evaluating, and improving scientific methodologies that have not yet been published by a SDO. The primary objective is to identify and promote viable discipline-specific standards for use by forensic laboratories and forensic laboratory accrediting organizations across the nation.

The OSAC includes three Resource Committees and five Scientific Area Committees (SACs) which are governed by a Forensic Science Standards Board (FSSB) that is authorized to supervise the organization and approve standards included in the OSAC Registry of Approve Standards. The FSSB is comprised of 17 voting members, of which 5 hold SAC chairs, 6 represent various forensic science associations (such as AAFS), 5 members from the research and measurement science communities at large, and 1 ex-officio member to break ties (OSAC 2014). The FSSB is responsible for overseeing the work performed by individual committees as well as participating in the international development of forensic science quality standards.

The Resource Committees consist of the LRC, the Quality Infrastructure Committee (QIC), and the Human Factors Committee (HFC). These critical committees provide their expertise to the OSAC by working with various committees and the FSSB to identify issues regarding human cognitive factors and legal ramifications of developed standards. The LRC, for example, collaborates with the legal community at large to provide guidance to the FSSB regarding legal issues that could affect the admissibility and acceptance of quality-assurance standards in forensic science.

The SACs are the foundational bedrock of OSAC. The five SACs cover broad forensic science topic areas with various subcommittees. The SACs and respective subcommittees are responsible for identifying standards that exist for forensic science service providers, thoroughly testing the standards and procedures for accuracy and reliability, and also producing standardized requirements for laboratory accreditation respective to the scientific discipline being investigated. The various subcommittees will investigate the status of their specific discipline's standards and procedures already in place and provide improvements and additional standards that will increase reliability and comprehension of the specific forensic science discipline. If the standard is approved by the SAC, it is then submitted to the FSSB for the final review to ensure the appropriate procedures were followed. By including a standard on the OSAC Registry of Approved Standards, the FSSB declares that the standard and its underlying methodology have been vetted by forensic practitioners, academic researchers, measurement scientists, and statisticians within the respective scientific community (OSAC 2014).

At the time of publication of this chapter, the OSAC Registry of Approved Standards contains 12 standards. Several dozen standards are under consideration for inclusion in the Registry in the near future.

6.8 The path forward for judicial and legal education in forensic science

The NAS Report states, "Lawyers and judges often have insufficient training and background in scientific methodology, and they often fail to fully comprehend the approaches employed by different forensic science disciplines and the reliability of forensic science evidence that is offered in trial" (NAS Report 2009, p. 27). Additionally, the Report states, "The fruits of any advances in the forensic science disciplines should be transferred directly to legal scholars and practitioners, ... members of the judiciary, and [other members of the justice system] so that appropriate adjustments can be made in criminal and civil laws and procedures, model jury instructions, law enforcement practices, litigation, strategies, and judicial decision-making." Further, judges and lawyers need to be better educated in forensic science methodologies and practices to better serve the administration of justice through credible forensic evidence.

Interdisciplinary knowledge sharing was a critical role of NCFS and OSAC in their development of more uniform and scientifically accurate forensic science disciplines. The legal consumers of scientific evidence may be far less knowledgeable about the accuracy of the procedures or methodologies used, as opposed to the scientists who are analyzing the evidence and forming expert opinions. With this in mind, the NCFS and OSAC worked diligently toward identifying scientific "problem areas" and creating a uniform set of practices to reduce confusion about forensic science and the applicability of such to both criminal and civil cases. Developments such as a forensic science curriculum for lawyers and judges are geared toward narrowing the gap between scientific methodologies and the practical understanding and use of scientific evidence. A more robust and uniform forensic science community would strengthen the credibility of forensic evidence and make the legal conclusions drawn from such evidence more readily determinable by judges, lawyers, and other forensic evidence consumers.

The American Bar Association Judicial Division[10] and The Journal of Criminal Law and Criminology (JCLC) held a symposium, *The Role of the Courts in Improving Forensic Science*, on 10 April 2015 (JCLC 2015). The symposium addressed the evidentiary issues that arise with forensic science evidence and expert testimony. Recommendations were made for judicial consensus of scientific reliability as well as a call for more legal and judicial education in the forensic sciences. During the ABA Annual Meeting on 4 August 2015 the House of Delegates adopted House Resolution 115 aimed at improving the courts' ability to evaluate forensic evidence, which provides:

> [T]he American Bar Association urges the National Commission on Forensic Science to develop a model curriculum in the law and forensic science, and to provide training in that curriculum for federal, state, local, territorial, and tribal judges.

In December 2015 the NCFS recommended that the Attorney General create and fund a curriculum that would explain and resolve various forensic science issues that are expected to arise in the courtroom (NCFS 2015c). The curriculum would facilitate both judges and lawyers in understanding and proffering forensic evidence. The NCFS (2015c) recommendation stated:

> Officers of the court see forensic issues in both criminal and civil settings. For that reason, it is essential that there be a curriculum that addresses both forensic science and legal issues as they will be presented in court—highlighting the disciplines and their limits and reasonably and neutrally presenting arguments that would support or challenge that evidence.

Recently, The National Judicial College (2015) announced several new courses that are geared toward "motivating judges to examine their role in the judiciary" and creating an environment that fosters discussion and finding practical solutions for judges. Resources such

---

[10] ABA Judicial Division (2015) *Resolution 115 Adopted*. (The House of Delegates is the policy-making body of the ABA. Any actions taken by the House of Delegates become official ABA policy.) http://www.americanbar.org/content/dam/aba/images/abanews/2015annualresolutions/115.pdf.

as the National Clearinghouse for Science, Technology, and the Law (NCSTL.org)[11] were developed to disseminate training, court decisions, commentary, scholarly publications, and other resources related to interdisciplinary forensic science topics and issues around the world.

The need for law and science interdisciplinary education is a global concern. In February 2015 a symposium was held in London, sponsored by The Royal Society, to bring together international researchers, academics and members of the judiciary to discuss developments in forensic science standards and reliability (Black and Daeid 2015). Topics discussed included cognitive bias, crime scene science, developments in various fields such as fingerprint identifications and virtual autopsies, as well as the legal framework for more robust and reliable forensic science evidence (Black and Daeid 2015). In addition, this meeting provided valuable insight into standards that are currently being developed and proposed a path forward for universal adoption and recognition of new standards (Black and Daeid 2015).

Following the two-day symposium, The Royal Society held a working group meeting at Chicheley Hall where a select group of 30 scientists, judges, and lawyers met to discuss research gaps in forensic science and identify fields in which additional research needs to be performed to ensure confidence in justice system outcomes (The Royal Society 2015). The focus was on strategic planning for the implementation of standards among forensic science service providers from the crime scene to the courtroom in order to effectuate a more capable and robust justice system around the world. As a result of The Royal Society Symposium and the work performed by the Chicheley Hall working group, in December 2015 the University of Dundee received a 10 million GBP grant to establish the Leverhulme Research Centre for Forensic Science (Isles 2015). The Centre Director is Professor Niamh Nic Daeid. Dame Sue Black, the former Director of the University's Centre for Anatomy and Human Identification (CAHID) and now Vice-Chancellor for Engagement at Lancaster University, was also instrumental in establishing the Centre.

---

[11] The National Clearinghouse for Science, Technology, and the Law (2016):
Homepage: http://www.ncstl.org
Accomplishments Database: http://www.ncstl.org/about/Accomplishments%20Archive.

While forensic sciences have seen challenges, the ultimate objective is the fair and effective administration of justice, which could be better served by an educated legal community regarding forensic testing and the reliability of the evidence being produced, especially in criminal cases in which an individual's liberty hangs in the balance (NAS Report 2009, pp. 27–28). The importance and effectiveness of expert testimony is a derivative of both the scientific methodology used as well as the lawyers' understanding the factors that the court will consider if admitting or rejecting the expert testimony. Continuing to educate judges and lawyers about the scientific foundations of expert testimony in the courtroom is essential to the success of improved forensic science standards. Lawyers and judges alike must better understand the complexities of forensic science methodologies, conclusions, and accreditation standards in order to adequately explain these factors to a jury charged with understanding and weighing expert testimony.

Acknowledgments

The author, Carol Henderson, would like to thank her Research Assistant, Ryan Swafford, Stetson College of Law, Class of 2017, for his valuable research and writing contributions to this chapter.

The author would also like to thank Kenneth E. Melson, AAFS President (2003–2004) and Distinguished Fellow, for his insightful comments on this chapter.

References

ABA Judicial Division and the Journal of Criminal Law and Criminology (2015). *The Role of the Courts in Improving Forensic Science Symposium.* ABA Judicial Division http://www.americanbar.org/groups/judicial/committees .html.

Black, S. and Daeid, N. (2015) The Royal Society Meeting: The Paradigm Shift for UK Forensic Science. London. https://royalsociety.org/~/media/events/2015/02/forensic-science/forensic-dm-programme910.pdf?la=en-GB.

The sections of this chapter that discuss *Daubert* is based on:Borenstein, J. and Henderson, C. (2015). Reflections on Daubert: a look back at the Supreme Court's decision. *Journal of Philosophy, Science & Law, Daubert* Special Issues 15: 1–4. http://jpsl.org/archives/reflections-daubert.

Butler, J. (2014). *Proceedings of the International Symposium on Human Identification*. Maryland: National Institute of Standards and Technology.

Cwik, C., Epstein, J., and Henderson, C. (2013). *Scientific Evidence Review: Admissibility and Use of Expert Evidence in the Courtroom*. Monograph No. 9. Illinois: American Bar Association.

Daubert v. Merrell Dow Pharmaceuticals, Inc. (1993) Supreme Court of the United States. U.S. Reporter, 509, 579–601.

FBI: National Press Release (2015). *FBI Testimony on Microscopic Hair Analysis Contained Errors in at Least 90% of cases in Ongoing Review*. Washington, DC: https://www.fbi.gov/news/pressrel/press-releases/fbi-testimony-on-microscopic-hair-analysis-contained-errors-in-at-least-90-percent-of-cases-in-ongoing-review.

Frye v. United States (1923). D.C. Circuit Court of appeal. *Federal Reporter* 293: 1013–1014.

General Electric Co. v. Joiner (1997). Supreme Court of the United States. *U.S. Reporter* 522: 136–155.

Haack, S. (2005). Trial and error: the Supreme Court's philosophy of science. *American Journal of Public Health* 95 (S1): S66–S73.

Herskovitz, J. (2016). *Influential Texas Panel Recommends Halt the Use of Bite-Mark Evidence*. Texas: Reuters.

Innocence Project (2016) Unvalidated or improper forensic science. http://www.innocenceproject.org/causes-wrongful-conviction/unvalidated-or-improper-forensic-science.

Innocence Project of Texas (2016). http://www.ipoftexas.org.

Isles, R. (2015). *University of Dundee: £10m Award to Establish Leverhulme Centre for Forensic Science at Dundee*. University News http://www.dundee.ac.uk/news/2015/10m-award-to-establish-leverhulme-centre-for-forensic-science-at-dundee.php.

Jasanoff, S. (1995). *Science at the Bar: Law, Science, and Technology in America*, 204–206. Cambridge: Harvard University Press.

Kumho Tire Co. v. Carmichael (1999). Supreme Court of the United States. *U.S. Reporter* 526: 137–159.

Morgenstern, M. (2016). *Daubert v. Frye – A State-by-State Comparison*. The Expert Institute, Blog https://www.theexpertinstitute.com/daubert-v-frye-a-state-by-state-comparison.

National Academy of Sciences Report (2009). *Strengthening Forensic Science in the United Stated: A Path Forward*. Recommendation 10, 11–28. Washington DC: National Academy Press.

National Commission on Forensic Science (2015a). *Ensuring That Forensic Analysis is Based Upon Task-relevant Information*. Human Factors Subcommittee http://www.justice.gov/ncfs/file/818196/download.

National Commission on Forensic Science (2015b). *Universal Accreditation*. Accreditation and Proficiency Testing Subcommittee.

National Commission on Forensic Science (2015c). *Forensic Science Curriculum Development*. Training on Science and Law Subcommittee http://www.justice.gov/ncfs/file/818206/download.

National Commission on Forensic Science (2016). *Recommendations to the Attorney General Regarding Use of the Term "Reasonable Scientific Certainty"*. Reporting and Testimony Subcommittee http://www.justice.gov/ncfs/file/816021/download.

NIST's Organization of Scientific Area Committees (2014) *Roles and Responsibilities*. http://www.nist.gov/forensics/osacroles.cfm.

NIST's Organization of Scientific Area Committees (2015). *ASTM: E2329-14 Standard Practice for Identification of Seized Drugs*. Registry of Approved Standards, Seized Drugs Subcommittee.

NIST's Organization of Scientific Area Committees (2016) *Registry of Approved Standards*. http://www.nist.gov/forensics/osac/osac-registries.cfm.

Palazzolo, J. (2016). Texas commission recommends ban on bite-mark evidence. *Wall Street Journal* http://blogs.wsj.com/law/2016/02/12/texas-commission-recommends-ban-on-bite-mark-evidence.

Reimer, N.L. (2013). *The Hair Microscopy Review Project: An Historic Breakthrough For Law Enforcement and A Daunting Challenge For the Defense Bar*. National Association of Criminal Defense Lawyers: The Champion https://www.nacdl.org/Champion.aspx.

The National Judicial College (2015) *The National Judicial College Announces 2016 Courses*. http://www.judges.org/the-national-judicial-college-announces-2016-courses.

The Royal Society (2015) The paradigm shift for UK Forensic Science – a further discussion. Working group meeting held at Chicheley Hall, Buckinghamshire. https://royalsociety.org/events/2015/02/forensic-science-satellite.

CHAPTER 7

Forensic odontology

Robert E. Barsley

American Academy of Forensic Sciences, New Orleans, LA, USA

7.1 Introduction

The field of forensic odontology, particularly the role played by forensic odontologists in identifying unknown human remains, has a long history in forensic practice. In addition to numerous anecdotal stories in which teeth played the defining role in proving the identity of a body, culminating with that of Paul Revere (silversmith, part-time dentist, and patriot) identifying the previously interred body from the Battle of Bunker Hill of his patient Gen. Joseph Warren; the first accepted recorded case in the USA was that of Dr. John Webster accused of an 1849 homicide in Boston, MA. The dismembered body of Dr. George Parkman was identified by comparing the recovered portions of the edentulous lower jaw with similarly recovered pieces of a dental prosthetic by Dr. Nathan Cooley Keep, the dentist who performed the dental treatment and had retained in his possession the plaster dental case upon which the dental prosthesis was fabricated. In the course of a sensational (for the times) trial lasting nearly two weeks and attended by thousands of spectators, another well-known dentist, Dr. William T. G. Morton testified for the defense in an effort to discredit the dental identification. Both practitioners were known for their pioneering work with the use of ether for surgical anesthesia. Dr. Keep would later become the founding Dean of the Harvard School of Dental Medicine. This case is remarkable in many ways—it was necessarily done without the use of dental radiographs (not "invented" until the late 1890s by the foundational work of New Orleans dentist

---

The Future of Forensic Science, First Edition. Edited by Daniel A. Martell.
© 2019 John Wiley & Sons Ltd. Published 2019 by John Wiley & Sons Ltd.

C. Edmund Kells). The case was also one of the first, if not the first, in which the identity of the body of the victim (Dr. George Parkman) was proven to a "reasonable degree" of certainty rather than absolute certainty that had been the required legal standard. The case also featured expert witnesses for the defendant. More than a century and a half later, the principle remains that an expert witness, including forensic experts, has the primary duty to present the truth—stating facts and the opinion drawn therefrom—and is not an "advocate" for his or her "side."

7.2 Roles of the forensic odontologist

From those humble beginnings, the field of forensic odontology/forensic dentistry has expanded in modern times to include identification services when multiple fatalities occur simultaneously such as in conflagrations, floods, and transportation accidents. The first well-documented occurred in Paris in 1897 with the Charité de la Bizarre fire in which local Parisian dentists, including Dr. I. B. Davenport form the USA, were able to assist in the positive identification of some of the more than 100 victims. Cuban-born dentist, Dr. Oscar Amoedo, chronicled the process in his 1898 book—*L'Art Dentaire en Medecine Legale*. The use of the teeth to estimate a dental or "biologic" age and compare those results with the chronological age have long played a role in dental treatment, especially when identifying and prescribing the onset of orthodontic treatment as well as deciding when (and even if) to remove unneeded teeth such as third molars and supernumerary teeth. In the forensic practice, the development of the teeth has long been used as a marker to determine the age at death, particularly in the young. As knowledge has progressed, teeth are now also used to assess the age of adult remains at the time of death and to determine if burials are "modern" or historic. For example, the presence of dental alloy/amalgam restorations in teeth is a sign that the individual could not have been alive prior to the mid-1800s, and the use of amalgam was not widely accepted in America until the 1890s. The use of silicate cements for anterior direct restorations began around 1910, whereas the presence of composite resin restorations moves that date forward by a half century to 1965.

Unfortunately, the lack of dental restorations is essentially of no value establishing the period in which the individual lived.

Similar to many professionals in today's world, dentists and the dental team are faced with recognizing (and reporting when appropriate) signs of abuse and/or neglect in children, adolescents, adults, and the elderly. Dental neglect can have wide-ranging effects on systemic health in all age groups, and for children, a high percentage of abuse involves injuries to the face and head areas—the realm of the practicing dentist. Similarly, some forensic dentists become experts in various fields of dental disease, diagnosis, and treatment—available to assist in litigation based on those issues, primarily professional liability in claims of negligence against other dentists. Many other professional disciplines (engineering and medicine, for example) have developed similar forensic experts/expertise.

The role of the forensic odontologist in the analysis and comparison of injuries attributed to the teeth, commonly referred to as "bitemarks" has been a topic of vigorous discussion for several years. Once again, the origins of the field have historical and apocryphal beginnings. An eleventh century English king who supposedly sealed and authenticated his written decrees by biting into the wax seal (as opposed to using a signet or simply signing them). History records the trials of suspected "witches" in which the accused was able to injure/torture the victim by causing "bites" to appear on various parts of the victim's body, often at will. In those cases, no expert was required to ascertain the origin or authenticity of the bite or link it to the "biter." The jury, the judge, or the receiver of the king's decree was given the leeway to decide for him or herself. The modern-day practice of bitemark analysis and comparison can fairly be said to have started in Texas in the 1950s. A burglar, in the process of robbing a grocery store, apparently took a bite from a block of cheese, leaving his "calling card" in the form of a bitemark in said cheese. The police investigating the crime asked a firearms expert to compare and measure the markings left by the criminal's teeth in the cheese with a similar block of cheese into which the suspect had voluntarily bitten. A local dentist was also consulted. Their independent opinions were that the suspect's teeth, as evidenced by the exemplar cheese, likely made the cheese left at the crime site. The case was upheld on appeal, and thus, bitemark analysis was deemed accepted by the court.

As additional cases were brought to trial, this case and subsequent cases that were unsuccessfully appealed based on the admission of bitemark testimony solidified the general acceptance of bitemark analysis and the ability of dentists to render expert bitemark opinions.

7.3   Current considerations

Forensic odontologists throughout the world have made great efforts to standardize and improve each of the fields of practice in which they are involved. In just one example, photographic techniques used in forensic dentistry were developed and perfected; in fact, the ubiquitous L-shaped scale so commonly used in all branches of forensic analysis today was first designed and produced in 1988 by an odontologist (along with a photogrammetrist/engineer) precisely to improve the analysis of bite injuries.

Over the last decade, much attention (and rightfully so) has been paid to the problem of improper convictions—based on withheld exculpatory evidence, outright forensic fraud, advances in forensic science and testing, mistaken eyewitness identification, coerced confession, and many other reasons. The rapid advances in DNA technology and testing have been at the forefront, and groups such as the Innocence Project have spearheaded the movement. Some of the cases of wrongful conviction have focused on bitemark analysis. Bitemarks as well as many other forensic techniques that can be generally classified as "identification" opinions have been subjected to increased scrutiny.

Some scientists studying the field refer to this as (drawing) a source conclusion. In its simplest sense, can one prove the assertion that items "A" and "B" originate from the same source? This could apply to a latent fingerprint—from the same finger; a fired bullet from the same firearm as another exemplar bullet, or two cartridge cases having been fired in the same firearm. Many forensic opinions dwell in this realm—the origin of two drug samples, the anthropological comparison of bony traits such as sinus patterns, dental identification based on the morphology of tooth structure, or dental restorative manipulations are other examples. Although some might argue that the simple choices of "Yes," "No," or "Insufficient material is available for analysis" are all that is needed, many argue that the stakes are so high that more information and therefore more certainty is required. Asking that question leads directly to several others—in many cases, the "ground" truth for a particular case can never be known as the circumstances cannot be duplicated and witnessed nor is there an empirical answer available. And for many of the questions posed, no data base or data warehouse exists to buttress the opinion or conclusion. For example, there is no collection of all the fingerprints in the world, no collection of all the firearm barrel rifling, or any database of the dental condition of all of the mouths in the world. How then should an expert express his or her conclusion? Some suggest a "likelihood" basis (although without availability of sufficient comparative data how can likelihood or odds ratio be calculated?). Experts in some fields have turned away from disfavored terms such as "a match" or "unique" to terms including "cannot be excluded" or "included as ___" or "excluded." Yet others are introducing terms such as "indistinguishable from" or "heretofore never encountered" (in this examiner's experience). Weighty questions of great concern to virtually all areas of forensic science.

Other issues that impact the practice of forensic dentistry in a manner unlike most other forensic disciplines is the educational path and professional or job opportunities associated with forensic odontology. Unlike the majority of forensic scientists and experts, forensic dentistry in the United States does not offer full-time employment. Most forensic odontologists are either faculty members of a dental college or are full-time practitioners of clinical dentistry in private practice. They are not part of a laboratory nor does anyone exercise supervision over their forensic practice. Although a pathway to certification in the field does exist, there is no requirement that one actually be certified before offering services. The educational path is also unlike that of forensic pathologists or forensic anthropologists, in many ways the closest parallels. After completion of dental school (and the issuance of a license to practice dentistry), no other formal education is required—contrast this to the forensic pathologist, who after graduating medical school must undertake a residency of several years in a specific medical field. In order to be a certified forensic pathologist, a residency in the field of forensic pathology as well as successfully challenging of the American Board of Forensic Pathology is required. Or the forensic anthropologist, who after receiving a bachelor's degree in physical anthropology must at a minimum earn a master's in anthropology to be even considered as an "expert." In order to challenge the American Board of Forensic Anthropology, an earned PhD in forensic anthropology is a requirement. In fact, virtually all forensic disciplines require additional classwork and specialized training. Masters and PhD degrees in forensic odontology are available in Europe and other countries, but until recently, no such advanced degrees in forensic odontology were available within the United States. In order to become certified in forensic odontology, a dentist must pursue additional classroom work and training, as well as demonstrate through casework expertise in forensic odontology. Most individuals challenging the American Board of Forensic Odontology require a minimum of five years to accrue these requirements. Of those deemed eligible to sit for the board, approximately two-thirds are eventually successful in the challenge. The American Board of Forensic Odontology and now the NIST Forensics—Organization of Scientific Area Committees (OSAC) are working to improve the practice of forensics across the nation. A lack of rigor in earlier years no doubt has some bearing on the poor marks accorded to bitemark analysis in cases from the 1980s and 1990s. The remainder of this chapter will examine the progress and future of areas in forensic dentistry in light of the preceding narration.

7.4   Identification by teeth

The "bread and butter" of forensic dentistry has always been the identification of unknown human remains. While fairly straightforward, there are complicating factors. Perhaps the biggest being the need to establish a putative identity through investigation in order to locate dental records for comparison. Unlike fingerprints and DNA, there are no data bases extant, which can be searched for possible matches leading to verification (or exclusion). In this author's opinion, despite advances in electronic health record-keeping, the specter of potential HIPAA violations and the lack of any centralized dental data storage or the clinical need for such a data base preclude development. That said, the advent of the electronic health record and the advances in all forms of digital imaging have made the retrieval of those records that do exist much easier and have improved the quality, availability, and transportability of the information as well. A dental practice can search for the name of a suspected victim (patient) at the push of a button. The search is more thorough than a manual search through written file folders in file cabinets and storage boxes would likely be, allows for variations in spelling, is not subject to the (former) purging of records of patients not recently seen, and is not affected by misfiling of patient folders. Because storage is no longer a function of physical space, there should exist a much greater chance that records of patients who were ever treated will be retained rather than destroyed. And that those records will be as "fresh" as the day they were recorded—no faded ink, no illegible handwriting, and a greater chance that all records of a single patient will be gathered in a single file rather than separate disparate files related to widely separated visits over time. But perhaps the biggest bonus will be that any radiographic images will also be present—again as pristine as the day they were acquired—no brown opaque analog film due to poor fixation/development, no misfiling of films, no failure to date films, no unnamed/attributable films, and no disposal or destruction of films due to space or destruction for recovery of silver products. One other benefit of the digital record will be that the contents can be completely transmitted anywhere in the world over the web instantly—no more waiting for courier pickup and delivery. Increasingly too, the future will allow for the reconstruction of the dental arch by the forensic odontologist as digital imaging and scanning replaces the clinical practice of obtaining dental models and impressions. The forensic odontologist of the future will have an actual exemplar of the oral cavity available in addition to the "historical" types of clinical and image data. Photographs of the teeth and of their clinical repair are also vastly easier to obtain (and of much improved quality) in the digital age—analog film-based photography was expensive and difficult in the past in contrast to today. All these advances will provide the odontologist so much more to compare to the unknown specimen. Similarly, he or she will have the same clinical advantages in gathering data form the postmortem specimen—better imaging, radiographic ability, and examination techniques. Today's best clinical dentists can restore teeth using techniques that yield clinical results that may escape the unaided eye of even a dentist without a very careful examination. Fillings whose margins are undetectable, crowns that resemble natural teeth in every respect, and dental implants replacing form and function—again almost natural appearing to the casual observer.

Digital record-keeping for the forensic dentist will be discussed a little later, but suffice it to remark at this juncture that just as in the retrieval of patient records from the dental office, the forensic dentist will be able to peruse his or her older entries and records when needed in much faster and broader ways to be certain that older cases are not inadvertently overlooked when partial or additional remains are discovered that might relate to a closed or "abandoned" case from years ago. The web has also broadened the search capabilities of investigative agencies when remains are found or missing persons' cases are considered. Improvement in the NCIC dental comparison algorithms and double-checking through the National Dental Image Repository (CJIS, FBI) have reinvented and made very useful this once underused modality. Last, but certainly not least in this area is the growing influence of the web through modalities such as The Doe Network and NameUS® (https://www.findthemissing.org/en), which afford the general public access to material to match potential missing persons with unclaimed or unknown remains. Curation by experts assists in moving cases with potential forward for definitive comparison and possible closure.

It is appropriate to move to the issues surrounding mass fatality incidents and the use of dental experts in verifying identity of the victims. Many of these issues have impact on the more routine identifications previously discussed. The forensic odontologist has long been an important resource for law enforcement when multiple victims result from an incident. This is particularly true when that incident results in damage to the remains that preclude the use of fingerprints to establish identity, a structure fire or a vehicle crash with fire, for example. Larger structures and large capacity vehicles complicate the case. The oral structures may suffer thermal damage, but in all but the most extreme cases, sufficient dental evidence remains to allow a competent forensic dentist to offer an opinion on the identification. The goal of course is to make identifications—"these remains are those of John Doe." However, especially in cases where the population of victims is considered "closed," that is, the inhabitants of a house, the driver and passengers of a vehicle, or even the passengers on an airplane (manifest), the forensic odontologist may only be able to state that there are no dental discrepancies due to a lack of either postmortem evidence or a lack of antemortem records/evidence. This nevertheless important finding may allow the investigators to combine the dental "findings" with other findings (personal effects, anthropology, scars/marks/tattoos, medical findings, etc.) to make an identification. Just as important, a single dental finding (a discrepancy between the antemortem records and the postmortem evidence) may easily be sufficient to exclude a particular set of remains from an identity—an example of a simple such case would be a set of remains with wisdom teeth present (not extracted) and antemortem proof (radiographs, etc.) that demonstrate that those teeth were removed prior to death. Similarly, a tooth in the remains that has not been restored (filled—crown, alloy, composite, etc.) is incompatible if ante-mortem records demonstrate that a particular tooth as having been restored. At least in today's world, people cannot regenerate teeth that were extracted nor can a person regrow tooth structure to replace a restoration.

As the number of victims mounts, the task becomes more complex, time-consuming, and beyond the ability of a single individual no matter how talented and dedicated to accomplish. Forensic dentists have long endorsed a team approach in these matters—teams that are trained and available to spring into action once alerted by the authorities. In the United States, there are county/metropolitan/regional teams, state teams, and even federal teams. The National Disaster Medical System (NDMS) under the auspices of the Department of Health and Human Services oversees the Disaster Mortuary Operational Response Teams (DMORT—one in each of the 10 federal regions) whose membership includes multiple specialists necessary to establish and operate a temporary morgue operation if the size of the disaster so dictates. DMORT has three complete morgues (equipment and supplies) palletized and ready for immediate delivery and deployment virtually anywhere in the world. Two are at airports, and one is loaded on semitrailers in the event air transport is not needed or not available. During the aftermath of Hurricane Katrina in 2005, two of these Deployable Portable Mortuary Units (DPMUs) were sent to Louisiana and Mississippi, personnel from all 10 federal regions were activated and manned the facilities as needed. The unit stationed in Louisiana remained in use until mid-February 2006.

While the concept of portable, deployable morgues predates NDMS, and the division of labor in the morgue and within the dental personnel—postmortem team, antemortem team, and comparison team—the equipment has undergone vast changes. What was once a completely handwritten exercise using analog film-based radiographs requiring careful record-keeping and filing and more importantly required the comparison team to have many of the original documents in their hands as they compared the deceased to the possible identities suggested by the antemortem records entered the computer age about 30 years ago. The Department of Defense, which suffers casualties in its ranks in peacetime and in war, through the US Army Institute of Dental Research developed software that could catalogue the ante-mortem and postmortem dental findings and perform crossmatching that would suggest the most likely matches for an odontologist's concentration. This program known as Computer Aided Post Mortem Identification (CAPMI) was a DOS-based. It was utilized with great success in several military disasters. As Windows®-based operating systems and Apple® systems gained in popularity, several other similar software were produced. A forensic dentist with an interest and background in computer coding developed the first version of WinID®, which gained popularity among American practitioners because of the simple graphical interface and a robust comparison scheme that allowed "plain language" filtering and produced several different sets of rankings each based on a slightly different comparison algorithm. DMORT adopted WinID. Similar programs were developed in other parts of the world, and this continues today.

Through use, problems were noted and changes were made. WinID was tweaked to allow a "marriage" between a particular digital radio-graphical scheme to allow the investigator to view radiographs without having to exit the program (at that time an annoying requirement in all programs). Digital radiography and portable, battery-powered hand-held X-ray generators became available allowing much greater flexibil-ity in acquiring postmortem radiographic images at a greatly improved speed. No film meant no delay for development and that the opera-tor could view the image within seconds, allowing the opportunity for additional and better exposures. This coupled with the elimination of the mechanical support arm and the need for electric power brought this capability directly to the autopsy table in disaster as well as routine forensic dental situations. Coupled with networked computers and centralized storage of all dental information, the ability to reach dental conclusions was greatly enhanced. The "dentists" were no longer the bottleneck at mass disaster morgue operations.

However, a few problems remained to be solved. Neither WinID nor any of the other programs could interface easily with any of the other disciplines in the morgue/identification operation, still requiring the transport of files (either printed or electronic) to the identification board. Simple questions that might be answered definitively by the exchange of a photograph ("the decedent had a gold font tooth" or "had a gap between his teeth") required a physical visit between investigators from two or more departments in the morgue operation. Separate files and separate protocols could hinder efficient (or even successful) backup operations. Software in other counties was developed to alleviate these difficulties—especially because of lessons learned from the December 2004 Southeast Asia Tsunami. In America, partly as a consequence of the World Trade Center Attack in 2001, the Office of the Chief Medical Examiner of New York City also tackled the problem, developing unified morgue operations software known as Unified Victim Identification System–Case Management System (UVIS-CMS) with a dental subcomponent known as UVIS Dental Identification Module (UDIM). The use of the dental software component is nearly intuitive, making entry of data simple and lessening the chance for error.

Error in entry can be deadly to results. Depending upon how "unforgiving" the dental comparison algorithm is, one single miskeyed entry can eliminate an individual from consideration, or place the correct record very far down in the list of suggested IDs. The question of just how much data are required to reliably suggest an identity is one that is currently unanswered. Historically, forensic dentists could be compared to "hoarders" of data—in the era of written only and film-based records coupled with the odontologist personally performing the comparison (no algorithm available), this is understandable. The slightest remembered or observed tidbit of data might be key to retrieving the two proper records—postmortem and antemortem. No one would want to miss that opportunity, and in many cases, once the remains were viewed, obtaining additional data from the remains was time-consuming in the least and difficult or impossible in some cases.

But computer comparison does not proceed in the same fashion as the human brain. One can assign the term "granularity" to the amount and depth of data collected (for the purpose of comparison). For example, is it more important to know that a tooth is merely restored as compared to what material is used in the restoration? Similarly, how important is it to know which surfaces are filled (consider a radiograph which depicts a restoration in the center of a lower molar), one cannot discern if the restoration is lingual or buccal, nor determine the material—but the fact that it is filled is highly germane in the comparison algorithm. It is important to remember that the forensic odontologist, not the computer, will perform the actual comparison and render the opinion. The software can only suggest which records should be the most fruitful in that effort and that every data point is retained in the antemortem and postmortem records regardless of whether or not it has a role in the initial comparison routine. Although the computer can process the information rapidly, obviously the more the data, the more involved the comparison. This leads to two questions—is there a great savings in resources such as computer time to be had with simpler data? Second, does the simpler data set have any appreciable effect on the results—is the most likely record still reported in the top three? Preliminary research seems to point toward to the utility of the "simple" data search.

One final question remains in his discussion of dental identification. How does the odontologist "prove" that his or her opinion is correct? Where can one find the so-called "ground truth"? This question arises in many forensic disciplines and is an ongoing bone of contention in bitemark analysis in the forensic odontology field as well. While dental misidentifications are thought to be extremely rare, this author is aware of at least one case where the "victim" surprised mourners at his own funeral by showing up a la Tom Sawyer style. I can state that in that case, the "dental ID" was performed by the coroner himself (not a dentist), and when confronted with the obvious error, he blamed it on the dentist who provided the antemortem dental records—of course, that begs the questions since that new individual then must have been the deceased victim, but he wasn't "dead" either. There have been other cases reported in which forensic odontologists have made errors, but they are as stated previously rare. This author is also aware of another case that has received great publicity in which a mother claims her son, the victim of prolific serial killer, was dentally misidentified as a victim and might still be alive. More than 10 well-trained and very experienced forensic odontologists have reviewed the case, and all have agreed that there are significant identifying features that support the opinion, in fact each of them, as well as the author, would not hesitate to sign such an opinion. The mother in this case cites irrefutable DNA evidence that excludes the remains as her son. But there are a few intervening factors. The initial dental ID was performed long before DNA identification was in use, and the remains in question were buried and exhumed some decades later. The path from the autopsy table to the grave contains pitfalls as well—the remains could have been mislabeled or misappropriated while in the coroner's custody before transfer for burial, the undertaker or the burial crew could have also mixed-up the remains/caskets. The exhumation may have been of the wrong gravesite. The DNA samples could similarly have been mixed-up. While the case has great import to those involved, it does highlight the earlier question—how can one be certain? No data base of human dentition exists. There is no data base of all the dental records located throughout the offices of the nearly 200 000 dentists in the United States. And this author doubts that either of the aforementioned data will ever exist. There are large dental practice groups, insurance companies, and even the Department of Defense that have access to large numbers of dental records; however, they are not organized in a manner that would allow comparison for identification purposes, nor would any of the principles be inclined to allow such to occur given the current state and federal privacy laws and regulations.

Research is needed in this field. Old studies demonstrated that identical twins have discernible differences in their respective dentitions. Those differences can only diverge as the individual's age, wear patterns on teeth, caries and restorations, extractions, injuries, etc. all lead to inevitable difference. Currently, the only data base related to this question is one known as OdontoSearch® (http://www.odontosearch .com/en/3.2/index.html) that contains dental information (excluding wisdom teeth) of more than 100 000 individuals. A forensic dentist can compare the postmortem dental findings of a case to that data base and receive a count of how many individuals have the same dental pattern (which can be expressed as an odds ratio or percentage). Although the results can be surprising, they do not offer any proof as to the veracity of the identity—certainly a prudent forensic dentist would take them into consideration based upon the degree of detail available in his or her case. As an example, in entering a mock case into the program, if only the information that teeth 19 and 30 have been extracted (and no other dental information is entered), then that dentition was common to over 19% of the data base population (nearly 20 000 dentitions). Refining the same search to include the additional information that all the remaining teeth that are present had not been filled ("virgin" in forensic odontology parlance), still yielded almost 250 similar dentitions.

7.5 Dental age assessment

Dental age assessment has gained popularity in the United States and worldwide in recent years. While many in the Unites States take for granted the ease with which one can prove (or have proven) their age (date of birth, DOB), in most of the world that is not so easy. Records are either not kept, not made available, or have been destroyed in many cases. Age is an important determinant in civil and criminal matters. In criminal matters, there is an age of "responsibility," the attainment of which renders the perpetrator subject to enhanced penalties. In administrative matters, such as marriage, voting rights, legal drinking age, age for issuance of a driver's license, age is an absolute requirement. Similarly, in some civil matters, the attainment of a specified age may impact a case. The development of the dentition, especially shedding (exfoliation) and eruption of the deciduous (baby) and permanent teeth, has long been recognized as a consistent and convenient means to assess or estimate age in children and adolescents. While studies have shown that variation exists between genders and population subgroups, the pattern is persistent, well recognized, and accepted with estimates having a range of 12–18 months or less in most cases. Documented studies are available and continue to be undertaken. However, once the age of 18 or so is reached, the dental findings and even the skeletal findings become less discriminatory and less reliable, and, as age increases, the ranges begin to approximate a decade or longer. While various tests and methods are available, many require the sacrifice of tooth, therefore, of little use in the living. One of the most popular uses in the United States recently has been to assess the likelihood that a detainee at a border crossing has attained the age of 18 years. If younger, the disposition of the case takes a different path from that of an adult, 18 years or older. There has been criticism of the use of dental age assessment if the assessment is based primarily on a panographic radiograph. Software has been developed to aid in the assessment. Guidelines, standards, and best practices are under development through the NIST–OSAC process. There is a large body of research that has been developed and is ongoing throughout the world in this field.

Another form of dental aging (besides age at death or during life, previously discussed) in the forensic world consists of estimating the historical time period from which the specimen originated. As discussed earlier, the mere presence and type of dental restorations may serve to date; however, the lack of dental restorations is not so enlightening. Radiocarbon dating (based on the decay half-life of Carbon 14 [^{14}C]) can be performed on teeth just as on other biological specimens that incorporate carbon into their structure. Additionally, due to atmospheric testing of nuclear devices in the 1950s and 1960s, yielding a greatly increased amount of ^{14}C to be available in the atmosphere and incorporated into the food chain, it is possible to determine a DOB estimate for individuals born after 1943.

7.6 Bitemarks

No doubt the most controversial aspect of forensic dentistry is bitemark analysis. Building upon earlier appellate court challenges, bitemark evidence became widely accepted and relied upon throughout the United States. However, not all bitemark analyses, nor all bitemark experts, performed at the highest levels demanded by a fair justice system. Although no appellate case to date has disallowed bitemark comparison as a valid forensic technique, there have been several instances in which specific bitemark-related testimony was deemed improper as well as cases in which additional nonbitemark evidence or reanalysis of previous bitemark analysis have resulted in verdicts being set aside, and in some cases, judgments of innocence have been handed down. In some of these cases, the expert testified improperly—linking bacteria found in a bite to a specific individual suspect, citing statistics with no factual basis, declaring that a suspect was the "biter" to the exclusion of all other individuals, etc. As previously discussed, this is another field in which the actual truth can never be known. It is complicated by many other factors as well. To what degree of reliability is the dental information of the biter's teeth and arch form transmitted and retained by the receiving substrate—in most cases, human skin? To what degree are dentitions "unique" in their morphology and is that at a level of measurement that can be ascertained and studied in bitemark cases? Is there a preferable method that should be used in the comparison? These are but a few of the questions that face the discipline. The reader is referred to a paper in the June 2018 issue of the *American Journal of Forensic Medicine and Pathology* that discusses many of these issues in depth.

Until recently, research on these and other questions has been relatively scarce. A National Institute of Justice-funded research project was concluded within the last decade, but has not been widely disseminated. Additional research using orthodontically treated arches, refrigerated porcine skin, and a "Procrustes-based" comparison scheme has been widely publicized, but many researchers and practitioners have voice dissatisfaction with the research model. Intuitional review boards (IRBs) at some universities have greenlighted studies using artificial jaws/biting devices on volunteers to begin to answer these questions. At present, research is underway to document and measure the forces involved in bite injuries and to study the effects of bites in living human volunteers. Of particular interest, here has been the fact that duplicating the force required to produce the types of injuries commonly encountered in assaults and homicides has been elusive. Other studies designed to explore the use of databases and digital capture of injuries and suspected biters' teeth have been conducted. As mentioned in identification, this is another field in which data bases are nonexistent. However, the wide spread use of digital devices and techniques to capture dental scans (rather than old-fashioned impressions and poured plaster models) does offer some hope, as deidentified dental arch data may become available for research use. One can certainly say that there is much room for improvement and great opportunities for research in this field. Again the NIST–OSAC process is laboring toward standards, guidelines, and best practices in bitemark practice.

7.7   Abuse and negligence

Two final fields of interest to forensic dentists are personal abuse, a field that impacts all dental practitioners and unfortunately numbers victims from all walks of life. Forensic odontologists are joining with pediatric dentists, dentists in long-term care facilities, abuse investigators, and physicians and nurses in combatting, documenting, and preventing this problem. The NIST–OSAC process is also tackling the problem and in conjunction with the American Dental Association is working to produce practice standards, guidelines, and best practices. The final field is that of dental negligence (malpractice) and related areas such as independent medical/dental examination (accidents for example) that routinely require testimony in articulating standard of care in the field or assessing the condition of an individual for courtroom purposes. While not linked necessarily to forensic practice, because many forensic dentists do testify and are familiar with the judicial system, many are drawn to this area—one shunned, at least on a voluntary basis by many dental practitioners in general.

7.8   Closing

In closing, it should be obvious that just as the case in other forensic disciplines, the field of forensic odontology remains involved in improving its knowledge base, its practitioners, its equipment, its techniques, and pursuing research to improve its foundations.

CHAPTER 8

Opportunities and problems faced in forensic pathology[1]

Edmund R. Donoghue[*]

Georgia Bureau of Investigation,Savannah, Georgia

The current state of forensic pathology in 2015 in the United States is fair to good. Medical examiner offices are currently meeting their needs for trainees in forensic pathology, and most trainees who want to work in the field are able to find employment. As we continue to recover from the Great Recession of 2008, some medical examiner systems enjoy adequate funding and infrastructure, while many other systems in the United States continue to face significant problems in funding for personnel, infrastructure, and technology. Within the time allotted for this presentation, your speaker would like to discuss selected problems faced by medical examiners at the current time.

8.1 Opportunity: radiology technology and computer imaging

Easy gains in quality improvement and documentation can be accomplished by distributing currently existing radiology and computer imaging technology to all medical examiner offices. The use of radiology is extremely valuable in locating and documenting bullets, foreign objects, fractures, medical devices, and personal effects on bodies.

[1]Presented at the Interdisciplinary Symposium of the 2015 Annual Meeting of the American Academy of Forensic Sciences.
[*]Past-President, American Academy of Forensic Sciences, 2005–2006.

The Future of Forensic Science, First Edition. Edited by Daniel A. Martell.
© 2019 John Wiley & Sons Ltd. Published 2019 by John Wiley & Sons Ltd.

Radiology is also very helpful in documenting abnormal fluid and gas accumulations in various areas of body cavities. On occasions when visual or fingerprint identification cannot be accomplished, dental and other diagnostic X-rays may establish or exclude identification by comparison with dental and clinical diagnostic X-rays taken before death.

A large majority of medical examiner offices have some access to radiology technology, whereas a few offices have limited or no access to this technology. In 2015, while some offices use only conventional cathode tube X-rays with film detection, others now have digital X-ray imaging that is viewed on computer monitors and stored and transmitted electronically. Some offices also have fluoroscopy with image intensification for special examinations, for example, precisely locating bullets. A few offices now have access to LODOX technology that can produce a full-body X-ray scan in 13 s with much lower radiation than conventional diagnostic X-rays. A very select group of medical examiner offices now have access to computerized axial tomography (CAT scan), a special imaging technology that produces cross-sectional images of the body using X-rays and a computer. LODOX and CAT equipment are many times more expensive than conventional medical X-rays. Additionally, for all types of radiology technology, the best images are produced by trained radiology technologists who understand exposure settings and know how to position the subjects correctly for examination. When radiology technology is utilized by autopsy assistants, the results may be of lower quality or unusable. Improved radiology technology and the personnel to operate, it would require increased funding for medical examiners.

8.2   Threat: dropping forensic pathology training requirement for anatomic pathology

Recently, there has been a discussion that the American Board of Pathology (ABP) might drop its requirement for hospital anatomic pathology residents to receive training in forensic pathology. Currently, the bulk of training in the performance of autopsies is being done in medical examiner offices. The elimination of this ABP requirement would virtually eliminate autopsy training for hospital pathology residents. Because hospital residents in anatomic pathology would no longer be trained in medical examiner offices, they would no longer be exposed to forensic pathology and could not be recruited as forensic pathology residents and future medical examiners. If this were to occur, medical examiners might have to establish training programs in autopsy pathology as well as forensic pathology to meet their needs for staff pathologist. Fortunately, at least for the present, the ABP has shown little inclination to take action on this idea, but medical examiners need to maintain vigilance.

8.3   Threat: maintenance of certification could see some forensic pathologists unemployed

Maintenance of certification (MOC) and recertification examination requirements for all physicians and specialties has become burdensome, and some states have attempted to require MOC as a condition of medical licensure. Prior to 1 January 2006, certifications issued by the ABP were granted for life and did not require further maintenance. As of 1 January 2006, all new primary and subspecialty ABP certificate holders are required to participate in the ABP MOC program. Continuing certification is contingent on participating in MOC and accomplishing all program interim requirements and deadlines during its 10-year cycle. If a certificate holder fails to meet reporting deadlines, a warning followed by expiration of the certificate occurs. The ABP's MOC program concentrates on four areas: (i) professionalism and professional standing, (ii) lifelong learning and self-assessment, (iii) assessment of knowledge, judgment, and skills, and (iv) improvement in medical practice. Certificate holders report progress in meeting their requirements every 2 years and must pass a secure examination during every 10-year cycle.

Physicians practicing full-time in forensic pathology should have no difficulty in passing the recertification examination in forensic pathology. They could, however, experience difficulty in passing the recertifying examination in anatomic pathology, which contains many items that are not seen in the daily practice of forensic pathology. Many medical examiner jurisdictions require the chief medical examiner to be certified by the ABP in anatomic and forensic pathology. Chief medical examiners who fail to meet all MOC requirements and pass both recertifying examination could find that they are no longer qualified to hold their positions.

8.4   Threat: standards are becoming increasingly detailed and rigorous

Standards for accreditation of medical examiner offices and autopsy guidelines are becoming increasingly detailed and rigorous particularly in the area of staffing requirements and the limits on the number of autopsies that medical examiners may perform. As originally devised accreditation and autopsy guideline were designed to establish the *minimum* requirements for medical examiner offices. As time progressed, the standards have been ratcheted down and become more exacting. Today's guidelines are becoming *ideal or aspirational* standards, that is, a standard we would all endeavor to reach under ideal conditions. These standards may be reachable with adequate staffing, infrastructure, and funding but may easily become unreachable when resources are scarce.

8.5   Threat: forensic: overregulation by federal government and other entities

Currently, the federal government and other entities are attempting to extend their influence over medical examiners. Having watched federal intervention in the clinical practice of medicine in the United States by statute, regulation, and funding for nearly 40 years, your speaker would suggest that the results have not been good for clinical physicians or patients. Forensic pathologists will need to be vigilant to avoid overregulation by the federal government and other entities.

8.6   Conclusion

In 2015, medical examiners face continuing problems in funding for vitally needed equipment, personnel, and infrastructure. In addition, they face additional regulatory burdens from their specialty board, accreditation organization, and the federal government.

CHAPTER 9

The future of forensic psychiatry and behavioral science

Richard Rosner

NYU School of Medicine, New York, NY

As one wit put it: "Prediction is always difficult, especially about the future." Given that caveat, the foreseeable future of forensic psychiatry and behavioral science will have at least two facets:

On the one hand, the current effort to advance neuroscience, for example, the US government's proposed $100 million Brain Research through Advancing Innovative Neurotechnologies (BRAIN) initiative is likely to advance our knowledge of the functioning of the brain and increase the scientific basis for our specialty.

On the other hand, as noted by Thomas Nagel in his recent book, *Mind and Cosmos*, certain basic problems are likely to remain either unaddressed or inadequately addressed. These problems include (i) the nature of consciousness, (ii) the relationship of the brain to the mind, and (iii) whether or not our subjective experience of "free will" is credible (Nagel 2012). Because our concept of personal responsibility (e.g., for criminal behaviors) is inextricably linked to those three issues, the impact of the anticipated scientific advances will be limited.

The Future of Forensic Science, First Edition. Edited by Daniel A. Martell.
© 2019 John Wiley & Sons Ltd. Published 2019 by John Wiley & Sons Ltd.

9.1 The BRAIN initiative

In April 2013, President Obama announced the launch of the BRAIN Initiative—a bold, new initiative focused on revolutionizing our understanding of the human brain.

The BRAIN Initiative is one of the Administration's "Grand Challenges"—ambitious but achievable goals that require advances in science and technology. Since the president announced the BRAIN Initiative, dozens of leading technology firms, academic institutions, scientists, and other key contributors to the field of neuroscience have answered his call and made significant commitments to advancing the initiative. Top neuroscientists also have developed a 12-year research strategy for the National Institutes of Health (NIH) to achieve the goals of the initiative (https://obamawhitehouse.archives.gov/share/brain-initiative).

The Brain Research through Advancing Innovative Neurotechnologies® (BRAIN) Initiative is part of a new Presidential focus aimed at revolutionizing our understanding of the human brain. By accelerating the development and application of innovative technologies, researchers will be able to produce a revolutionary new dynamic picture of the brain that, for the first time, shows how individual cells and complex neural circuits interact in both time and space. Long desired by researchers seeking new ways to treat, cure, and even prevent brain disorders, this picture will fill major gaps in our current knowledge and provide unprecedented opportunities for exploring exactly how the brain enables the human body to record, process, utilize, store, and retrieve vast quantities of information, all at the speed of thought (www.nih.gov/science/brain).

9.2 The law and the human mind

Embedded in the law, especially in criminal law, is a de facto set of assumptions about human beings and human psychology. With the exception of "strict liability" cases (Wachs 2008), crimes entail an actus rea and a mens rea, a guilty act and a guilty mind. To be guilty of a crime, it is not sufficient to have broken the law, that is, to have engaged in an actus rea. The perpetrator of a criminal act must also substantially possess the ability to know what he is doing and substantially have the ability to appreciate the wrongfulness (criminality) of his action, that is, to have mens rea. To be criminally responsible for one's acts, the law assumes the existence of a conscious mind, a mind that is capable of rationally deliberating and freely choosing to engage in a course of conduct.

Forensic psychiatrists and forensic psychologists may assist the court in both criminal and civil issues involving the evaluation of mental states of persons. The BRAIN initiative and the neurosciences generally address anatomical and physiological matters. Almost no one doubts that there are important associations and correlations between brain states and mental states. However, the exact causal mechanisms by means of which brain states may produce mental states is unknown.

9.3 Correlation is NOT causation

There is no doubt that brain events are often correlated with mental events. The ongoing puzzle is the nature and significance of those correlations. An example of the difference between correlation and causation is found in the fact that the beating of African tom-tom drums during a solar eclipse has always been followed by the restoration of the sun.

> Whenever there is a reliable correlation between A and B, there are three possible causal explanations. A caused B, B caused A, or A and B were both caused by something else. In addition, it could be that A and B are actually the same thing even though they do not appear to be (like water and H_2O, or the morning star and the evening star).
>
> *(Blackmore 2005, pp. 21–22)*

9.4 Theories of consciousness

There are many theories that purport to explain the phenomenon of consciousness (Taylor 1992, pp. 9–34).

One such theory is known as interactionalism. " … while the mind of a person is not a physical thing, events that transpire within it sometimes have causal consequences or effects within the body.

Conversely, although the body of a person is clearly not a mental or nonphysical thing, the events that occur within it, particularly within the nervous system and brain, sometimes have causal consequences or effects within the mind or consciousness" (Taylor 1992, p. 18).

A second such theory is epiphenomenalism. " ... according to which mental entities, such as thoughts, images, ideas, and feelings, never enter as causes into any physical processes, and hence never act upon the body or any parts of it, yet are sometimes, if not always, the effects of bodily processes, particularly those within the nervous system" (Taylor 1992, p. 25).

Yet a third theory is materialism. " ... I might just be the totality of my bodily parts, suitably related and all functioning together in the manner expressed by saying that I am a living body, or a living, material animal organism" (Taylor 1992, p. 11).

A fourth theory is idealism. " ... idealists denied the existence of matter, maintaining that all bodies, including one's own, exist only as ideas in some mind" (Taylor 1992, p. 26)

A fifth view is double-aspect theory. " ... suggested that there is really only one kind of substance, and that we call 'mind' and 'body' are simply two aspects of this" (Taylor 1992, p. 26).

A sixth theory is parallelism. " ... it has been supposed that mind and body, being different substances, never act upon each other, but the histories of each are nevertheless such that there seems to be such a causal connection" (Taylor 1992, p. 26).

A seventh theory is occasionalism. " ... maintained that all of one's mental life is caused, from moment to moment, by God, who sees to it that this mental life is in close correspondence with what is going on in the body" (Taylor 1992, p. 26).

An eighth theory is pre-established harmony. " ... parallelism is wrought by God, who, in creating a person, arranges in advance that the mental and physical histories should always be in close correspondence without interacting ... " (Taylor 1992, p. 26).

9.5   The hard problem of consciousness

A popular version of materialism is functionalism, that is, that mental states are functions of brain states. To analogize: driving is a functional state of an automobile, and, it is theorized, consciousness may be a functional state of the brain. However, we know exactly how the engineering of an automobile enables it to be driven. We have no such understanding of how the anatomy and physiology of the brain might produce the subjective experience of consciousness. That ongoing riddle is often referred to as "the hard problem of consciousness."

"How can a physical brain, made of purely material substances and nothing else, give rise to conscious experiences or ineffable qualia? How do subjective experiences arise from objective brains?" (Blackmore 2005, pp. 1–16).

What is it like to be you? The answer entails a description of your subjective conscious experience. To be conscious means that there is something that it is like to be you (or someone else). Anything of which one cannot ask "What is it like to be that?" is not conscious.

Subjective experience is what consciousness is about. It is the experience of how things seem to be to you, as contrasted with objectivity.

Qualia are the subjective experiential qualities that you have, for example, the aroma of a rose, the colors of a rainbow, the soft feel of fur, and the taste of pineapple. These are unique to consciousness.

9.6   Consciousness and the failure of the physical sciences

The physical sciences can describe organisms like ourselves as parts of the objective spatiotemporal order—our structure and behavior in space and time—but they cannot describe the subjective experiences of such organisms or how the world appears to their different particular points of view. There can be a purely physical description of the neurophysiological processes that give rise to an experience and also of the physical behavior that is typically associated with it, but such a description, however complete, will leave out the subjective essence of the experience—how it is from the point of view of its subject—without which it would not be a conscious experience at all.

(Nagel 2013)

Colin McGinn argues that because we know the mind by internal first-person ("I") introspection, whereas we know the brain by external third-person ("he, she, it") observation, so that there is no shared basis for both kinds of information, it is intrinsically impossible to understand how physical brains and immaterial minds are related. "The fact is that no point of view permits us to integrate the observable features of the brain with its invisible conscious features" (McGinn 1996).

9.7   The problem of free will

> Whether we have control over how we act, and what this control requires and involves, and whether and why it matters that we have it.
>
> *(Pink 2004, p. 2)*

One of the ongoing disputes is whether or not free will exists, whether it might merely by an illusion. "Causal determinism is the claim that everything that happens, including your own actions, has already been causally determined to occur. Everything that happens results from earlier causes ... " (Pink 2004, p. 13).

Nonetheless, the subjective experience that (at least some of) your actions are "up-to-you," that you are free to decide which of alternative actions (or inactions) in which to engage, is a conviction deeply held by most people (Taylor 1992, pp. 35–53). "Our natural assumption is that our having control of how we act depends on our actions not being causally determined in advance by factors outside of our control—by factors such as the environment we were born into, the genes we were born with, the desires and feelings that come over us beyond our control. This assumption that we so naturally make is called incompatibilism, so-called because it says that freedom is incompatible with the causal predetermination of how we act by factors outside our control. ... Libertarianism about freedom of action combines Incompatibilism with the further belief that we do actually possess control over how we act" (Pink 2004, p. 13).

The law presupposes that we are responsible for our actions because we have freely chosen them. Generally, if we had no choice, if we were not free to act or not, then we were not responsible for our bodily action. " ... human freedom is also presupposed in our legal systems, when courts punish people and hold them legally to account for what they have done. ... punishment is fair only if the person punished was in control of their actions—if it really was up to them whether or not to act as they did" (Pink 2004, pp. 9–10).

9.8 The bottom line

The thrust of the argument made by Professor Thomas Nagel in *Mind and Cosmos* is that the physical sciences, including neuroanatomy, neurophysiology, and the neurosciences generally, are not able to explain subjectivity. It is not that we lack information or technical skills that might become available in the future. Rather, it is that the material domain of the neurosciences is intrinsically so different from the nonmaterial domain of personal subjectivity (e.g., consciousness, the nature of the relation of the brain to the mind, and free will) that the former can never explain the later. The gap between brain states and mental status will remain unbridgeable. Thus, the advances in neuroscience from the BRAIN initiative and similar projects will not obviate the concepts embedded in the law, for example, mens rea, malice aforethought, responsibility.

In so far as can be discerned, the future of Forensic Psychiatry and Behavioral Science will be marked both by fresh discoveries in the neurosciences and by continuity in the questions that the law will pose to practitioners.

References

Blackmore, S. (2005). *Consciousness*. Oxford: Oxford University Press, pp. 1–16, 21–22.

McGinn, C. (1996). *The Character of Mind*, 2e, 46. Oxford: Oxford University Press.

Nagel, T. (2012). *Mind and Cosmos: Why the Materialist Neo-Darwinian Conception of Nature Is Almost Certainly False*. Oxford: Oxford University Press.

Nagel, T. (2013). The Core of "Mind and Cosmos", *The Stone, The New York Times* (18 August).

Pink, T. (2004). *Free Will*. Oxford: Oxford University Press, pp. 2, 13, 9, 10.

Taylor, R. (1992). *Metaphysics*, 4e. Englewood Cliffs, NJ: Prentice Hall, pp. 11, 18, 25, 26, 9–34, 35–53.

Wachs, R. (2008). *Law*. Oxford University Press, pp. 48, 50–51, 58, 132.

CHAPTER 10

The future of forensic document examination

John L. Sang[1], Linton A. Mohammed[2] and Carl R. McClary[3]

[1] *Forensic Document Examiner, Nassau County, NY, USA*
[2] *Forensic Document Examiner, Forensic Science Consultants, Inc.,Burlingame, CA, USA*
[3] *Forensic Document Examiner Bureau of Alcohol, Tobacco, Firearms, and Explosives,Atlanta, |GA, USA*

Document examination evidence and testimony has been used in US Courts for over 100 years, and courts around the world for longer than that (more specifically handwriting comparison evidence and testimony). Forensic document examiners (FDEs), sometimes known as handwriting experts, are offered by attorneys to the courts on either side of an issue. Various jurisdictions around the nation have rules that are used to qualify examiners at court/trial. The various courts have additional rules regarding the acceptance of questioned and known documents into evidence.

Before we address cutting-edge research and technologies, we have to lay a foundation for what the disciple of FDE is and the scope of work of a FDE.

10.1 What is a forensic document examiner (FDE)?

FDEs conduct many types of examinations beyond just handwriting comparisons. The American Society of Testing and Materials International (ASTM) standard defined this work in the **Scope of Work of Forensic Document Examiners in E444-09**. On January 4,

The Future of Forensic Science, First Edition. Edited by Daniel A. Martell.
© 2019 John Wiley & Sons Ltd. Published 2019 by John Wiley & Sons Ltd.

2012 Scientific Working Group for Forensic Document Examination (SWGFDOC) sent out a letter that they are now mandated to "create, prepare, and publish standards guide lines for their constituents in their forensic community" Prior to this they forwarded their draft standards to ASTM. SWGDOC.org SWGDOC standards that describe in general, the duties of FDEs, also referred to as questioned document examiners. (QDEs), document examiners, or document analysts and examination procedures.

The **Job Description**. The FDE makes scientific examinations, comparisons, and analyses of documents in order to

1. establish genuineness or nongenuineness, or to expose forgery, or to reveal alterations, additions, or deletions,
2. identify or eliminate persons as the source of writing,
3. identify or eliminate the source of typewriting or other impressions, marks, or relative evidence, and
4. write reports or give testimony, when needed, to aid the users of the examiner's services in understanding the examiner's findings.[1]

FDEs refer to those who meet minimum training standards as defined formerly in the ASTM E2388-11 and, currently, the SWGDOC Minimum Training Requirements for FDE and also required by the QD section of the American Academy of Forensic Sciences (AAFS), the American Society of Questioned Document Examiners (ASQDE), associated regional organizations, and those individuals certified by the American Board of Forensic Document Examiners (ABFDEs).[2]

> Document examinations play an important role in the criminal justice process. The issue of genuineness of documents presents itself in nearly all forgery prosecutions, kidnappings involving ransom notes, confidence games and embezzlements. " . . . ." Apart from these, however, questioned document evidence may occur in nearly every other type of crime as well, including homicides, thefts, robberies, arson, burglaries, etc.
>
> *Moenssens and Inbau (1978, p. 464)*

---

[1] ASTM International, 100 Barr Harbor Dr. PO Box C-700 West Conshohocken, Pennsylvania 19428-2959, United States Scope of Work of Forensic Document Examiners in Standard Guide E444-9. This scope of work is also available as a Scientific Working Group for Document Examiners (SWGDOC) standard and can be accessed at www.swgdoc.org.

[2] Not all individuals who claim to be FDEs received the appropriate minimum training and followed the published standard guidelines, or adhered to the ethical standards talked about here today.

In addition, document examiners work on civil cases and a good number of examiners are not connected with law enforcement. Civil cases usually involve will contests, disputed contracts, and patents.

> The function of the document examiner is not limited to determining whether some specimen of handwriting or typewriting has been made by a suspect individual. He is also concerned with other facets of forgery detection. Among them are the authentication and dating of documents; the decipherment of erased, obliterated, charred, and water damaged documents; and the restoration of faded or chemically erased writings; indented writings; suspected substitution of pages; the study of paper watermarks and of printing, copying and duplicating processes; and the detection of alterations.
>
> *Moenssens and Inbau (1978, p. 464)*

Riordan et al. (2012), did an excellent job at providing the origins of QDE starting on page 14 of Chapter 9. These foundations provide context for our chapter on looking to the future so with Bill's permission, I have provided it here.

10.2 Origins of questioned document examination

Disputes concerning the authorship and authenticity of documents have been occurring since ancient times. Laws in ancient Rome provided for the acceptance of expert testimony concerning documents (Huber and Headrick 1999). In 1562, the English Parliament declared forgery to be a statutory offense, and in 1684, "comparison of hands" was ruled to be "good evidence in cases of treason." A significant legal step occurred in 1762, when a British court ruled that handwriting is identifiable (Levinson 2001).

Early courts sometimes relied on "recognition witnesses"—someone who was familiar with a given writer's handwriting and would testify to it in court (Huber and Headrick 1999). The use of someone with a specialized skill in comparing known standards with questioned handwriting gradually became the more accepted practice. The first case in English-speaking courts in which a specially qualified witness testified was *Goodtitle d. Revett v. Braham* in 1792, in which a direct comparison between questioned and known writings was conducted rather than reliance on recognition. In this case, two experts were admitted, their special qualifications being that they had experience as inspectors of franks (Huber and Headrick 1999).

While there is little written history of document examination in America until the late nineteenth century, there are records of court decisions, particularly after 1800, which show that there were individuals testifying about handwriting identification; names of the experts, however, do not seem to have been recorded until after 1870 (Hilton 1979; Levinson 2001). An 1808 Louisiana code (code of 1808, p. 306, art. 226) stated that, in resolving a question of authorship, a questioned signature "must be ascertained by two persons having skill to judge of handwriting" who would then determine authorship based on comparing it to known writings. Just a few years later in the Louisiana case of *Sauve v. Dawson, 2 M.R. 203 (1812)*, a signature on a promissory note was compared to an appeal bond executed by the defendant and determined to be genuine (Louisiana Supreme Court 1854).

These early cases conformed to rules derived from English common law that decreed that questioned writings could only be compared to known writings that were already in evidence in a case. Decisions in Massachusetts in 1814 and later in Connecticut and Vermont removed this restriction and allowed the admittance of other writing samples (Hilton 1979), which greatly expanded the potential to pursue handwriting comparisons as a form of evidence in cases.

The profession of document examination gained significant recognition in the mid-nineteenth century with a case involving the Junius Letters. These were a series of letters written and published around 1770 that discussed many controversial issues of the time dealing with liberty, politics, and government in England. The author used the pen name Junius, and much speculation occurred for decades regarding the true identity of Junius. Charles Chabot, one of the earliest practitioners in the field of QDE, concluded from a handwriting examination that the author was Sir Philip Francis (Chabot and Twisleton 1871). His clear and thorough presentation of his evidence and conclusions helped document examination gain acceptance in the English legal system (Levinson 2001).

Legal decisions of the 1880s and 1890s affirmed the importance of handwriting evidence and the use of experts, saw ink examination accepted as testimony and also the first testimony on typewriter identification in 1893 (Levinson 2001). Several early examiners wrote books on QDs that were published in the 1890s: *A Treatise on Disputed Handwriting* (1894) by William Elijah Hagan, *Manual for the Study of Documents* (1894) by Persifor Frazer, and *Ames on Forgery* (1899, 1900) by Daniel T. Ames.

10.3   Albert S. Osborn and the formation of the American Society of Questioned Document Examiners (ASQDE)

Albert S. Osborn (1858–1946) is widely considered to be the founder of modern document examination. He began a career as a penmanship instructor at the Rochester Business Institute in New York. In those days, it was common practice for an attorney to consult a penmanship instructor to examine and draw an opinion about disputed handwriting cases. Osborn is recorded to have been working as a document examiner in 1887, and began publishing articles on the topic (Hilton 1979; Levinson 2001; Osborn 1910).

In 1910, he wrote *QD*, a classic work that brought together the fundamental principles of the field formulated over the past century, and broadened the scope of QDE to include typewriting, ink, and paper examinations. Through his writings, lectures, and testimony, handwriting identification began to gain wider acceptance in the courts and in society (Hilton 1979; Huber and Headrick 1999).

In 1929, he revised his classic work, *QDs*, and throughout his career wrote several other books and many articles on document examination and expert testimony. He also wrote extensively about courtroom procedures, expert testimony, court presentation, and legal decisions, publishing *The Problem of Proof* in 1922 and *The Mind of the Juror* in 1937 (Hilton 1979).

Also during this time period, document examination gained additional attention and acceptance through the writings of Professor John H. Wigmore of Northwestern University School of Law, who also wrote the introduction for several of Osborn's books. Wigmore, a noted authority on American Evidence Law, contributed greatly to the acceptance of expert testimony and document examination as a forensic science around the turn of the century (Hilton 1979; Huber and Headrick 1999).

In 1913, Osborn and another examiner, Elbridge W. Stein, met together to discuss topics dealing with handwriting examination, and to initiate a program for the exchange of ideas and research. This was followed by a larger gathering in 1914 at Osborn's residence in Montclair, New Jersey. These meetings were by invitation only, and gradually expanded and occurred annually. Membership required annual attendance, as well as active participation; participants presented a paper each year that was then discussed by the group. In 1942, Osborn and 14 other prominent examiners formally organized as the ASQDE, with Osborn as the first president (Levinson 2001; The Origin of the ASQDE n.d.).

Up until the 1920s and 1930s, document examiners worked in the private sector, with many having started as penmanship instructors, though other professions included bankers, lithographers, engravers, court clerks, and police officers (Hilton 1979; Huber and Headrick 1999; Levinson 2001). The 1920s and 1930s saw the opening of the first federal, state, and local crime laboratories in the United States. In the 1930s, two examiners were known to be doing QD work for the federal government in the Bureau of Standards and the Treasury Department (Hilton 1979). The first major police Questioned Documents Laboratory in the United States was opened in Chicago in 1938.

10.4   Ordway Hilton and the formation of American Academy of Forensic Sciences (AAFS)

The First American Medico-legal Congress, which was the precursor to the Academy of Forensic Sciences, was addressed in January 1948, by George Swett, a document examiner with the US Postal Inspection Service. The Steering Committee Meeting convened in October 1948 by Dr. R. B. H. Gradwohl at the Hotel Pierre, New York City, was attended by Document Examiners Ordway Hilton and Albert D. Osborn.

In 1950, the AAFS adopted a Constitution and By-laws setting up seven sections, and James Clark Sellers, charter member and first vice president of the ASQDE, became the first QD section Chairman. Presenters at the Third Academy meeting, in 1951, included QDE, and in 1952, Section Chairman Ordway Hilton began correspondence that influenced the development of an active QD Section within the AAFS. Largely due to the efforts of Chairman Ordway Hilton, assisted by Secretary David J. Purtell, section membership number requirements were met and QDs held its first section meeting with a program of technical papers at the AAFS meeting in 1953. At this time, forensic sciences were advancing as crime laboratories were growing. Initially, most members of the ASQDE were leery of meeting and sharing their collected knowledge with examiners outside of the society. However, Donald Doud, who was a well-respected private examiner and member of the ASQDE, worked along with Ordway Hilton to convince the society members to support the AAFS. Ordway Hilton, David J. Purtell, and Donald Doud were the real pioneers who worked to form the QD Section. Thanks to these pioneers, government as well as private FDEs from various areas of the country, including members of the ASQDE, eventually joined and supported the AAFS QD Section. Historically, there has been a very prolific group of FDEs that possessed dual membership in both the AAFS and the ASQDE (Hilton 1979; ABFDE n.d.).

Mr. Hilton earned degrees in mathematics and statistics at Northwestern University, which had a scientific crime investigation laboratory within its law school. The Northwestern Laboratory was developed toward the end of the 1920s. Northwestern Law Professor Emeritus Fred Inbau was instrumental in the transition of the Northwestern Laboratory to the City of Chicago for its police department in 1938. The same year, Ordway Hilton who had pursued a career in FDEs, was chosen to be the first document examiner for the Chicago Police Department Crime Laboratory by Professor Inbau. Mr. Hilton became highly regarded and internationally recognized for his achievements in the field of FDEs. He was the author of a leading textbook and a monograph on pencil erasures and published over 90 articles for scientific and legal journals and lectured at law schools across the country. Ordway Hilton was the president of the AAFS in 1959 and president of the ASQDE in 1960 and was awarded the honor of Distinguished Fellow by the Academy. In recognition of his outstanding contributions to the field of FDEs, he was awarded the first the AAFS QD Section award, an award that is in his name, the "Ordway Hilton Award." Mr. Hilton, like his fellow QD Section pioneers, was also a diplomate of the ABFDE.

10.5 Questioned documents and the formation of the International Association of Forensic Sciences (IAFS)

The first International Association of Forensic Sciences Meeting in conjunction with the International Meeting in Forensic Immunology, Medicine, Pathology and Toxicology, was held in London, England, in 1965. This meeting was attended by members of the AAFS QD Section as well as members of the ASQDE. From the inception of the IAFS, FDEs has been one of the forensic disciplines represented at the Association's triennial meetings. The IAFS has fostered the international exchange of information in forensic sciences including research, and standard practices.

10.6 Key issues

10.6.1 Certification

In the 1970s, the need to identify qualified professionals in the forensic science disciplines lead to serious discussions regarding the establishment of certification boards within the United States. The Department of Justice became aware of the need to support the development of these professional boards. "The Department of Justice has funded, through the Law Enforcement Assistance Administration (LEAA), a program of certification in forensic sciences. This program is administered under the auspices of the AAFS. Certification boards in forensic toxicology, forensic odontology, forensic psychiatry, forensic anthropology, and forensic document examination have already been constituted" (Crown 1989).

10.6.1.1 Certification and the American Board of Forensic Document Examiners, Inc. (ABFDE)

The AAFS Committee on Certification was formed in 1974 and Dr. Kurt M. Dubowski was selected to chair this important committee that proposed and established certification programs in forensic sciences. In 1975, the Report of the Committee on Certification was presented to Dr. David A. Crown, President of the AAFS and Chief of the CIA's QD Laboratory. Following the report, the Forensic Science Foundation obtained a Law Enforcement Assistance Administration (LEAA) grant and helped establish the American Board of Forensic Document Examiners, Inc. The ABFDE was incorporated in the District of Columbia in 1977 with John J. Harris, President, James J. Horan, Vice President, James H. Kelly, Secretary and Maureen Casey Owens, Treasurer.

"The objectives of the Board are to establish, enhance, and maintain standards of qualification for those who practice forensic document examination and to certify, as qualified specialists, those voluntary applicants who comply with the requirements of the Board." Each candidate's personal education, professional education, training, experience, and successful completion of a formal three-part examination process, is the basis of certification (ABFDE n.d.).

> By 1980, more than one hundred experts have been certified by the ABFDE and granted diplomate status. The Questioned Document Board certification is somewhat similar to the Board Certifications conferred in the medical field to various types of specialists. In other words, it is a formal recognition of expertise by a high quality professional board, though by no means a compulsory or legally required recognition for licensure or conduct of business.
>
> *Crown 1989.*

10.6.2 Standardization

10.6.2.1 AAFS QD task group on opinion terminology

Thomas V. McAlexander, Jan Beck, and Ronald Dick, the members of an AAFS QD Section task group on opinion terminology, presented a paper entitled, "Committee Recommendations: The Standardization of Handwriting Opinion Terminology" at the 1990 AAFS annual meeting that was published the following year as a letter in the *Journal of Forensic Sciences*. The terminology (a nine-level scale) was accepted by the QD section of AAFS and by the ABFDE. The positive and negative terminology in the scale allows for the expression of various levels of certainty.

A need for "qualified" conclusions exists because of possible limitations in the questioned and/or known materials that can preclude a definite conclusion. Restrictions effecting QDs such as copying processes, limited clarity, brevity, and physical damage as well as limitations in known documents such as insufficient comparability, limitations in amount, disguise, and a lack of contemporaneous samples are common factors that hamper examinations and may lead to a "qualified" conclusion. The use of the term "probable," "probably," or "probability" used in the standard is addressed by the authors: "probability in handwriting opinions is not a statistical measurement but a measure of the examiner's confidence, based on scientific principles and experienced judgment, that the opinion rendered is correct. This is true because probability relates to qualitative as well as quantitative processes" (McAlexander et al. 1991).

The acceptance of the standardized handwriting opinion terminology was a major accomplishment within the field. It required a great deal of interactive debate and compromise among the FDEs throughout the country. Prior to this standard terminology, the wide-spread diversity of expressions limited the possibility for a clear, uniform understanding of "qualified" conclusion terms used in the field.

"Committee Recommendations: The Standardization of Handwriting Opinion Terminology" was the basis for ASTM E1658 Standard Terminology for Expressing Conclusions of Forensic Document Examiners, which was drafted and passed by the ASTM E30.02 Questioned Document Subcommittee.

10.6.2.2 ASTM International

ASTM International (formerly, the American Society for Testing and Materials) is one of the largest voluntary standards development organizations in the world. In 1970, ASTM E30 Committee on Forensic Science was established with the goal of developing standards in the forensic sciences. The E30.02 Questioned Document Subcommittee was established to develop standards in forensic document examination. ASTM procedures accommodate the process of the drafting of standards; the balloting of the draft to the E30.02 Subcommittee (which considers the votes of the ballots at an annual meeting); the balloting of the draft to the E30 Committee; the final evaluation and vote by both the E30.02 Subcommittee and E30 Committee (at the following annual meeting); and the request of the Committee on Standards for publication approval. The E30.02 standards had been developed by the diligent work of task groups.

10.6.2.3   Scientific Working Group for Questioned Documents

The Technical Working Group for Questioned Documents (TWGDOC) began in 1997 and was one of the first of the technical working groups in the forensic sciences. TWGDOC met in various Washington, DC area locations. This national group, composed of FDEs from the private sector and from federal, state and county laboratories, was renamed the Scientific Working Group for Questioned Documents (SWGDOC) in 1999. After 1999, meeting space was offered to SWGDOC as well as other scientific working groups at the FBI Academy in Quantico, Virginia.

SWGDOC made the determination to publish through ASTM International where draft documents are reviewed by a variety of forensic disciplines. SWGDOC subgroups, usually composed of five to seven individuals, develop drafts or updates that are vetted through other subgroups before submission, as drafts, to ASTM International E30.02 Questioned Documents Subcommittee.

> The mission of SWGDOC is to assemble representatives from the forensic document examination community in order to define the scope and practice areas of the profession; standardize operating procedures, protocols, and terminology; consolidate and enhance the profession of forensic document examination; and promote self-regulation, documentation, training, continuing education, and research.
>
> *SWGDOC n.d.*

In summary, Forensic Document Examinations are more than handwriting examinations (Riordan et al. 2012). It includes examinations of

- Office machines
- Paper and ink for differentiation and dating
- Obliterations, alterations, indentations examinations
- Counterfeit document examinations.

FDEs work frequently with other experts to conduct comprehensive examination of documents and evidence. This includes DNA, ink, paper, plastics, latent prints, bomb residue/components, and digital data collection (as an example of this is at NYPD, John Sang had a patent authentication case that involved photocopies, a computer, and a fax machine). He suggested they bring Allen Brill of their New Digital Imaging Section with the legal team to Rome, Italy, and Allen ended up conducting the bulk of the examinations.

So experts from different disciplines working together get us closer to finding the truth or facts about the documents (history) and other evidence.

John Sang has been fortunate to have specialized in terrorist cases for seven years while in the QD Section of NYPD's Crime Laboratory. At one point, there were over 10 FDEs in that section. John had at his disposal a vast resource of over a 100 chemists and other experts to help resolve the cases at hand. While John was a supervisor of the QD Section, he recruited people from other Laboratory Sections—Chemistry, Serology, and Criminalistics—so that he could expand the knowledge base of the section. In fact, John's father, a FDE, was recruited by the Document Section from the Laboratory Chemistry Section and went on to be the assistant director of the United States Postal Service Laboratory, New York.

10.7   Standards of practice

Two important operational standards for Document Examiners are the following:

SWGDOC's Scope of work of a Forensic Document Examiner (FDE), formerly ASTM E444-09, that I described earlier on and SWGDOC's Minimum Training Requirements for Forensic Document Examiners, formerly ASTM Standard E2388-11.

This standard provides the minimum requirements and procedures that should be used for the fundamental training of FDEs. The procedures outlined within are grounded in the generally accepted body of knowledge and experience in the field of FDE. By following the requirements and procedures in the standard, an appropriate trainee can acquire the scientific, technical, and other specialized knowledge, skill, and experience required to reliably perform the work of a FDE.[3]

The Scientific Working Group for Forensic Document Examination (SWGDOC) develops standards and guidelines for the field of FDE. SWGDOC is composed of private examiners and government examiners from local, state, and federal laboratories throughout the United States. SWGDOC began in 1997 as a TWGDOC, was renamed SWGDOC in 1999, and was reorganized in 2001. From 2000 to 2012 SWGDOC published their standards through the ASTM. In 2012, SWGDOC stopped publishing their standards through ASTM and began self-publishing their standards as is the practice for nearly every other SWG group. For additional details view their website at www.swgdoc.org.

SWGDOC standards are available to all free of charge as SWGDOC continues to update and enhance extant standards and generate new ones. As in the past, SWGDOC standards are based on the efforts of numerous examiners from the public and private sectors along with individuals in the legal and academic worlds. The broad range of input and thorough peer review of this process produces the highest quality standards—standards that can be used to produce reliable examination results.

SWGDOC Standard for Scope of Work of Forensic Document Examiners

SWGDOC Standard for Test Methods for Forensic Writing Ink Comparison

SWGDOC Standard Terminology for Expressing Conclusions of Forensic Document Examiners

SWGDOC Standard for Writing Ink Identification

SWGDOC Terminology Relating to the Examination of Questioned Documents

SWGDOC Standard for Examination of Mechanical Checkwriter Impressions

SWGDOC Standard for Examination of Dry Seal Impressions

SWGDOC Standard for Examination of Fracture Patterns and Paper Fiber Impressions on Single-Strike Film Ribbons and Typed Text

SWGDOC Standard for Physical Match of Paper Cuts, Tears, and Perforations in Forensic Document Examinations

---

[3] ASTM International, 100 Barr Harbor Dr. PO Box C-700 West Conshohocken, Pennsylvania 19428–2959, United States Minimum Training Requirements for Forensic Document Examiners formerly ASTM Standard E2388-11. This standard is also available as a Scientific Working Group for Document Examiners (SWGDOC) standard and can be accessed at www.swgdoc.org.

SWGDOC Standard for Examination of Rubber Stamp Impressions

SWGDOC Standard for Examination of Handwritten Items

SWGDOC Standard for Indentation Examinations

SWGDOC Standard for Nondestructive Examination of Paper

SWGDOC Standard for Examination of Altered Documents

SWGDOC Standard for Minimum Training Requirements for Forensic Document Examiners

SWGDOC Standard for Examination of Documents Produced with Liquid Ink Jet Technology

SWGDOC Standard for Examination of Documents Produced with Toner Technology

SWGDOC Standard for Examination of Typewritten Items

SWGDOC Standard for Preservation of Charred Documents

SWGDOC Standard for Preservation of Liquid Soaked Documents

SWGDOC Standard for Use of Image Capture and Storage Technology in Forensic Document Examination.[4]

The Organization of Scientific Area Committees (OSAC) was formed in 2015 and the Forensic Document Examination is one of the founding committees. The Physics/Pattern Evidence SAC comprises the following disciplines:

- Questioned Documents
- Blood Stain Pattern Analysis
- Friction Ridge
- Firearms and Toolmarks
- Footwear and Tire Tread.

The subcommittee on FDE will focus on standards and guidelines related to the discipline, including

1. source of handwriting,
2. source of machine-produced documents, typewriting, or other impressions and marks,
3. materials and devices involved in the production of documents,
4. genuineness and alterations,
5. preservation and/or restoration of legibility,
6. documentation and reporting, and
7. training and competency.

---

[4] The twenty-one (21) SWGDOC Standards are available at www.swgdoc.com.

It is anticipated that the OSAC will play a key role in future standards development for the discipline, and the AAFS Academy Standards Board, ASB, process is already being utilized in the revision of the previously published standards.

10.8   The Daubert standard and FDE

FDE was one of the first forensic disciplines to seriously address the Daubert challenges, beginning in 1995 with *US v. Starzecpyzel*, the first FDE challenge. The judge ruled that FDE expertise was a technical or specialized knowledge, and at that time was outside the scope of Daubert.

We advised the leaders of the Academy and explained in a short period of time Daubert was going to affect all of the disciplines at the Academy. Following the 1999 Supreme Court decision of *US v. Kumho*, which decided that the *Daubert standard* also applied to *expert testimony including* scientists and nonscientists. This early exposure to the new Daubert standard allowed us to get a head start and prepare ourselves for what was to come. An FDE Daubert Group was established to educate the courts and seek funding for continued research studies. We received funding for our research and were able to make remarkable strides forward in our research.

"The turning point for forensic document examination occurred in a *Daubert* hearing in March 2002, *United States v. Prime*". "------" The basic theory of handwriting individuality was supported by an ongoing research involving computer measurement of handwriting features as well as several published studies involving document examiners' ability to consistently distinguish the handwriting of identical twins. The studies of Dr. Moshe Kam not only provided the profession's error rate but also convinced the judge that the Kam results superseded any purported statistical data previously based on flawed proficiency test conducted in the 1980s. Perhaps most compelling was the judge's observation that if forensic handwriting testimony was excluded based on an overly rigid application of *Daubert*, then a criminal defendant would be prevented from presenting contradictory, exculpatory evidence in his or her defense.

The 9th Circuit Court affirmed the *Prime* decision on appeal in 2004, and conspicuously noted the fact that all six circuits that had previously addressed the admissibility issue of forensic handwriting examination had also affirmed its reliability.

Kelly and Lindblom (2006)

Today, our discipline has successfully responded to 47 Federal *District Court* Daubert challenges, with no Federal Appellate Court-level exclusions. That is out of about 24 appellate cases to my knowledge, not a single QD case has been cited in the Wrongful Conviction study. To this day, we track relative Daubert challenges to determine how the courts are applying Daubert and the Law, allowing us to keep up with the changing times.

We are not attorneys and are not claiming to be. The law and science (forensic science) are two different disciplines. The forensic scientist's responsibility is to perform good ethical science and assist the trier of fact with his or her examination results. Each state and legal jurisdictions may have different rules and interpretations. I will address "The Daubert Rule" from an FDE or layperson's perspective.

The Daubert Rule came out of the case "*Daubert v. Merrell Dow Pharmaceuticals,* 509 U.S. 579 (1993). The issue: Is plaintiff's evidence of animal studies and unpublished re-analysis of previously published human studies scientifically reliable to prove that Bendectin, an anti-nausea drug for pregnant women, causes birth defects in babies?"

On appeal, the U.S. Supreme Court reversed the Court of Appeals for the Ninth Circuit and set forth certain factors to be considered by judges reviewing scientific evidence and remanded the case back to the Ninth Circuit for further consideration.

The US Supreme Court established the following standards:
1. The Judge is a "gatekeeper" of evidence under Rules 104a and 702.
2. In order to determine if proffered scientific evidence or testimony is "reliable" as evidence the Judge must determine if the evidence is "ground(ed) in the methods and procedures of science."
3. That inquiry envisioned by FRE 702 is "flexible."
4. The characteristics of scientific methodology distinguishes science from other fields of human endeavor.

5. Before admitting scientific, technical, or other specialized knowledge a court should ascertain whether the evidence or testimony of a theory or technique:

   a. Can be or has been **Tested** (falsified or refuted)?

   b. Was it subjected to **Peer Review and Publication**?

   c. Is there a known or potential **Rate of Error**?

   d. Is it "**Generally Accepted**" in the relevant scientific community?

AAFS 58th Annual Meeting, Workshop #24 How Frye and Daubert have Changed the Presentation of Criminalistics and Questioned Documents in Court. Chair Joseph J. Maltese, JD Co-Chair John L. Sang, MS. Expert Testimony: Scientific, Technical and other Specialized Evidence, presentation by Joseph J. Maltese, JD, 2/21/2006.

10.9   How FDE meets Daubert

All of the professional scientific studies to date involving forensic handwriting examinations have validated the proficiency of FDE expertise in handwriting examinations. Forensic scientists always must keep in mind that the judge is the gatekeeper of evidence and testimony and a judge, upon review of qualifications, may not admit an examiner.

The members of the FDE discipline have addressed the Daubert factors as follows:

10.9.1   Standards

As mentioned previously, questioned documents has utilized ASTM as its publishing body for standards and now by the Scientific Working Group for Document Examiners (SWGDOC), for nationally recognized standards. The standards can be accessed at www.swgdoc.org.

Certification has been available since 1977 by ABFDE. It determines whether a FDE candidate has satisfied the minimum standards of competency. Certification is based upon the candidate's personal and professional education, training, experience, and achievement, as well as on the results of an extensive three part examination process.

ABFDE is accredited by the Forensic Specialties Accreditation Board (FSAB).

The ABFDE is sponsored by the *Canadian Society of Forensic Science*, the *American Society of Questioned Document Examiners*, the *Southwestern Association of Forensic Document Examiners*, and the *Southeastern Association of Forensic Document Examiners*, and also is recognized by the *Questioned Document Section of American Academy of Forensic Sciences*, the *International Association for Identification*, the *Midwestern Association of Forensic Scientists*, and the *Mid-Atlantic Association of Forensic Scientists*. The ABFDE is the only certifying body that can claim such sponsorship and recognition.

The **American Society of Crime Laboratory Directors/** Laboratory Accreditation Board (ASCLD/LAB) is an accrediting board of peers that determines whether a forensic laboratory complies with specific standards.

ASCLD/LAB includes the inspection and accreditation of forensic document laboratory sections.

10.9.2 Error rate/reliability

Although no critical error rate in any forensic field has been substantiated, numerous studies conducted since the early 1990s have confirmed that FDEs are significantly more reliable than nonexperts at reaching correct conclusions in the examination of handwriting, hand printing, and signatures, both natural and disguised.

In fact, Kam * found that nonexperts are six times more likely to identify the wrong writer than an expert (see Kam et al. 1994, 1997 *, 2001; Kam and Lin 2003; Found 2002). Dr. **Moshe Kam** of Drexel University, Distinguished Professor, Data Fusion Laboratory, Electrical and Computer Engineering Department studies found that laypeople are six (6) times more likely to identify the wrong writer than experts. Dr. Kam in 2014 was appointed Dean of Newark College of Engineering.

So if a handwriting case goes to trial without a document examiner, it may not be advantageous for the attorneys' client.

Dr. Kam started studying FDEs relative to handwriting expertise prior to our first Daubert examination. He has handwriting studies published from 1994 to 2008 and published many in the *Journal of Forensic Sciences*, a publication of the AAFS.

Kirsten Singer, ABFDEs president, writes in ABFDE News that Dr. Kam became involved in the QD profession, as he puts it, "by accident." In 1991, he submitted a proposal for an FBI project to computerize handwriting searches. At the time, one of his students suggested that they ask the handwriting experts how they do what they do. Dr. Kam suggested he just go to the library and bring back all the papers that describe the proficiency of document examiners. The student returned with only one, the "Exorcism" paper by Risinger, Denbaux, and Saks that detailed how few studies existed in the proficiency of forensic handwriting examination.

As Dr. Kam explains, " . . . . It became quite important for us to do this (conduct proficiency studies). In other words, if we are going to try to code it, as significant expense and time, and if students are going to write a thesis on this and so on, we better test to see that we get information from a reliable source."

Dr. Kam proceeded to conduct the first pilot study in 1992 and 1993, which led to the large-scale study published in 1997, "Writer Identification by Forensic Document Examiners" followed by other peer reviewed studies, all of which showed that proficiency testing results by FDEs and laypersons are statistically different (therefore an expertise exists); error rates of FDEs are far smaller than those of a layperson; and monetary incentives to laypersons do not improve their performance.

10.9.3 Testing of basic principles

One of the basic principles of forensic handwriting examination is that no two persons with mature, individualized handwriting will share the same combination of handwriting characteristics. Studies that support this principle are the following:

a. Studies of the handwriting of identical twins. There are at least three published studies, one involving 50 sets of identical twins (Beacom 1960), one involving 58 sets of identical twins (Gamble 1980), one involving 95 sets of twins (Boot 1998).

   All of these works came to the same conclusion that with a sufficient amount of handwriting samples, it was always possible to distinguish the handwriting of identical and fraternal twins.

b. The United States Secret Service (USSS) and The Federal Criminal Police Office of Germany (BKA) maintain databases known as the Forensic Information System for Handwriting (FISH), with the USSS version containing handwriting specimens from a combined 110 000+ writers. To date, no two writers have been found to have the same combination of handwriting characteristics.

c. The Center of Excellence for Document Analysis and Recognition (CEDAR), at the State University of New York (Srihari et al. 2002), conducted a study "for the purpose of establishing the individuality of handwriting. The work was motivated by U.S. high court rulings that require expert testimony be backed by scientific methodology. Since handwriting had not been subjected to such a study, we decided to undertake this endeavor. A data base was built representing the handwriting of 1500 individuals from the general U.S. population. The sample was made representative of the U.S. population by stratification and proportional allocation. The population was stratified across different genders, age group and ethnicities. Individual discriminability was established by using a machine learning approach where some samples are used to learn writer characteristics, and other samples are used to test the learned models. Based on a few macrofeatures that capture global attributes from a handwritten document and microfeatures at the character level from a few characters, we were able to establish with a 98% confidence that the writer can be identified. Taking an approach that the results are statistically inferable over the entire population of the U.S., we were able to validate handwriting individuality with a 95% confidence. By considering finer features, we should be able to make this conclusion with a near 100% confidence." "----" "our work has employed handwriting features similar to, but not exactly the same as those used by document analysts in the field. However, the objective analysis that was done should provide the basis for the conclusion of individuality when the human analyst is measuring the finer feature by hand."

d. A study published in 2009 utilized a group of writers from the same New York neighborhood and elementary school and concluded that

FDEs were able to ascertain inter-writer variation and identify significant characteristics toward identification. The examiners rendered definitive conclusions of authorship with an overall accuracy score of 98%. Durina and Caligiuri (2009).

e. Srihari et al. conducted research "On the discriminability of handwriting of twins" 2008 *JFS*, **53**(2) where he wrote "The distinctiveness of each person's handwriting has long been intuitively observed. Methods have been developed for a human expertise of handwriting matching over many decades (Louisiana Supreme Court 1854; Hilton 1979; Huber and Headrick 1999; Levinson 2001; ASTM Standard E444 2009). Yet there is a need for studies in the quantitative assessment of the discriminative power of handwriting particularly for the acceptance by the courts of evidence provided by FDEs. In a previous study of handwriting individuality (Chabot and Twisleton 1871), we reported on the discriminability of handwriting of a diverse population from across the United States. The present paper reports on a complementary study of the discriminatory power of handwriting when the population consists of a cohort group consisting of twins. Both the previous study and the current study are based on automated methods for handwriting comparison. The current study uses algorithms that are updated with respect to the types of handwriting features that are computed." From the Summary and Discussion of the research Srihari writes "The discriminability of the handwriting of twins is a useful measure of the individuality of handwriting. Results of automated handwriting verification using handwriting specimens from twins and nontwins have been presented. When no rejection is allowed, the verification error rate using different content, half page writing is 12.6% for twins and 3.15% for nontwins. By allowing rejection, the verification error rate can be reduced to less than 4% and less than 0.5%, respectively. When comparing identical twins with fraternal twins with different writer testing cases, the difference of error rates shows that handwriting of identical twins is more similar than that of fraternal twins."

The fact that error rate with twins is higher than with nontwins is probably consistent with biometrics that is based purely on physiological factors such as fingerprints and DNA. Distinguishing between the handwriting of twins is harder than that of nontwins because twins are more likely to have the same genetic and environmental influences than others. The results for nontwins are also consistent with the results of a previous study of the general population. The error rate for nontwins was about the same as that of the previous study, although the textual content of the pair of documents used in verification was different, the textual passages were smaller (half pages), and the characters used in the matching process were automatically determined (rather than manually, thus introducing some errors).

Comparison with human performance, on half-page of writing tests, shows that system performance is better than that of nonexpert humans. From a system design point of view, this is encouraging in that reaching human performance has been the goal of most work in artificial intelligence. With further system improvements, system performance can hope to reach the performance of QDEs. The current system is based on a set of simple features. The use of better features, for example, those with a cognitive basis such as the ones used by QDEs, and higher accuracy classification algorithms should further decrease the error rates. As expert human performance has been shown to be significantly better than that of lay persons, many sophisticated improvements are likely to be needed to reach the higher goal.

1. Osborn (1929).
2. Robertson (1991).
3. Bradford and Bradford (1992).
4. Huber and Headrick (1999).
5. Hilton (1993).
6. Srihari et al. (2002).

For additional reading on the subject as it relates to QD see *AAFS News*, July 2010, Vol. 20, Issue 4. Reliable, Relevant and Valid Forensic Science: Eleven Sections-One Academy, The AAFS Questioned Document Section Plays a Principal Role in the Substantiation of the Validity and Reliability of Forensic Document Examination. Source: Carl R. McClary, BA Questioned Document Section Chair.

10.9.4 Peer review and publication

Numerous articles that address forensic document examinations have been published in the following peer-reviewed journals:
Journal of Forensic Sciences
Journal of the American Society of Questioned Document Examiners

Forensic Science International
Canadian Society of Forensic Science Journal
Journal of Forensic Identification
Journal of Police Science and Administration
Science and Justice formerly (*Journal of the Forensic Science Society*)
Journal of Criminal Law and Criminology.

10.9.5   General acceptance in the forensic community

Forensic handwriting examination was one of the founding sections of the AAFS and has had its own national organization, the ASQDEs, since 1942. It is an expertise that has been provided in all major law enforcement organizations, and numerous state and local agencies.

Forensic document sections are also included in the following multidiscipline organizations:

International Association of Identification (IAI)
Mid-Atlantic Association of Forensic Scientists (MAAFS)
Midwestern Association of Forensic Scientists (MAFS)
Northeastern Association of Forensic Scientists (NEAFS)
Forensic Science Society (FSS) (Charter Member)
Canadian Forensic Science Society.

Forensic document examination is or has been a part of the curriculum taught at the following schools:
* The George Washington University
* Michigan State University
* John Jay College
* National University (San Diego)
* University of Alabama at Birmingham
* University of New Haven
* University of Central Oklahoma
* University of Illinois at Chicago
* Oklahoma State University.

John Sang besides teaching FDE Courses at John Jay College and University of New Haven have taken FDE Courses at John Jay College and Georgetown University.

Since 2006, Oklahoma State University has offered a Graduate Certificate in Questioned Documents program. The Certificate program may also be taken as a part of OSU's Master of Forensic Sciences degree.

10.10　Research in FDE

10.10.1　Neuroscience

A study of dynamic variables by van Gemmert (1996), van Galen (1984), Hardy, and Thomassen (1996) provides an example of a neuroscientific approach to understanding disguised handwritten text. Dynamics is concerned with the study of forces and torques and their effect on motion. Disguised writing is the writing of a person who deliberately attempts to alter the elements of one's own writing (Huber and Headrick 1999). In this study, several dynamic variables (captured using a digitizer tablet and a pressure-sensitive pen) were assessed, and it was found that disguised handwriting was bigger than normal handwriting and had increased duration.

There was no significant difference in disfluency between genuine and disguised handwriting (as measured by comparing the frequency of pen acceleration changes between the populations). They found pen pressure increased from 1.08 N in normal to 1.35 N in disguised (free style) and pressure was higher in cursive script than print script. Slant was not found to be a discriminatory feature that was later supported by Coupland (2004) who demonstrated that the angle value test and angle measurements were both unreliable as a means of discriminating between the genuine and disguised signatures of the same writer.

Mohammed et al. (2011) conducted a kinematic study of genuine and disguised signatures. Kinematics studies the motion of objects without reference to its causes. They found that with genuine signatures, there were significant differences between styles for size, velocity, and pen pressure, and there were significant differences between genuine signatures and at least one of the unnatural signature conditions for all parameters. For velocity and size, these changes with condition were dependent on style. Changes with condition for the other parameters were similar for the three styles. This study shows that there are differences among natural signature styles and disguise behaviors that may be relevant in forensic signature examinations.

Caligiuri et al. (2014) conducted a study on the kinematics of signature writing in healthy aging. The primary purpose of this study was to systematically examine age-related changes in signature kinematics in healthy writers. Signatures were recorded using a digitizing tablet, and commercial software was used to examine the temporal and spatial stroke kinematics and pen pressure. Results indicated that vertical stroke duration and dysfluency increased with age, whereas vertical stroke amplitude and velocity decreased with age. Pen pressure decreased with age. They found that a linear model characterized the best-fit relationship between advanced age and handwriting movement parameters for signature formation. Male writers exhibited stronger age effects than female writers, especially for pen pressure and stroke dysfluency.

Highly programmed skilled movements are executed in such a way that their kinematic features adhere to certain rules referred to as minimization principles. One such principle is the isochrony principle, which states that the duration of voluntary movement remains approximately constant across a range of movement distances; that is movement duration is independent of movement extent. The concept of isochrony suggests that some information stored in the motor program is constant, thus reducing the storage demands of the program. In a study of the isochrony principle, Caligiuri et al. (2012) found that genuine signatures adhered to the isochrony principle, whereas simulated signatures did not.

van Gemmert and van Galen (1996) looked at the dynamics of genuine and forged[5] handwriting. They found that forgers were successful in copying the spatial aspects of handwriting such as size, slope, and general appearance. However, from the kinematic data, the investigators found that forged handwriting, in comparison to the genuine model, exhibited slower speeds, longer reaction time, and was generated by more frequent but smaller force pulses. They found pen pressure to be higher in the forgeries, but the peak values of pen pressure in the genuine samples were higher. Their results further indicated that that the stiffness of the writing limb is greater when imitating another person's style, and they considered that this may be a mechanism the forger uses to combat stress. They concluded that simulated script is widely different from authentic script in the dynamic domain. The van Galen (1984), van Gemmert et al. (1996), and van Gemmert and van Galen (1996) studies were among the first to demonstrate

---

[5] The words forged and simulated are defined as an attempt by one person to copy another person's signature or handwriting style. Forgery is a legal term and is not normally used by FDEs who prefer the term *simulation*.

the value of quantitative analyses of pen movement dynamics during handwriting.

Mohammed et al. (2015) in a kinematic study of signatures found that stroke duration, velocity, and pen pressure were found to discriminate between genuine and simulated signatures regardless of the simulator's own style of signature or the style of signature being simulated. However, there was a significant interaction between style and condition for size and jerk (a measure of smoothness). The results of this study, based on quantitative analysis and dynamic handwriting features, indicate that the style of the simulator's own signature and the style of signature being simulated can impact the characteristics of handwriting movements for simulations. Writer style characteristics might, therefore, need to be taken into consideration as potentially significant when evaluating signature features with a view to forming opinions regarding authenticity.

In a study that looked at dynamic characteristics of signing behavior, Franke (2009) found that velocity, pen pressure, and pen lifts or pen stops were not sufficient to discriminate between genuine and forged signatures. The author concluded that "Only the local, inner ink-trace characteristics as well as variations in ink intensity and line quality can provide reliable information in the forensic analysis of signatures." However, this study only comprised a very limited number of subjects.

10.10.2   Eye tracking

Dyer et al. (2008) evaluated the performance of 8 FDEs and 12 control subjects at identifying signatures as either forgeries or the disguised writing of a specimen provider. Subject eye movements and response times were recorded with a Tobii 1750 eye tracker during the signature evaluations. Using a penalty scoring system, they found that FDEs performed significantly better than control subjects. An analysis of eye movement search patterns by the subjects indicated that a very similar search strategy was employed by both groups, suggesting that visual inspection of signatures is mediated by a bottom up search strategy. However, FDEs spent greater than 50% longer to make a decision than the control group. The findings are suggestive that for some stimuli FDEs can discriminate between forgeries and disguises, and that this ability is due to a careful inspection and consideration of multiple features within a signature.

Another eye-tracking study was conducted by Merlino et al. (2014). This research empirically explored the reliability, measurement validity, and accuracy of established FDE procedures using a multimethod, multidisciplinary approach. They investigated basic issues of validity and reliability in signature comparison tasks.

One phase of the study, conducted with 49 FDE and 43 lay participants as a comparison group, encompassed four different experimental eye-tracking protocols, and was conducted under controlled laboratory conditions using Tobii T-60 model binocular eye-tracker systems. The signature stimuli were prepared to capture several different signature features, such as signature complexity, signature type (text-based, mixed, or stylized), and type of process used to create the signature (genuine, disguised, traced, or freehand simulation) that might be encountered as part of the FDE caseload.

Eye-tracking and self-report results revealed high construct validity for the formal index used by FDEs to evaluate the authenticity of handwriting. High convergent validity was also demonstrated via the two methods, indicating that the results obtained by eye-tracking and self-report revealed similar findings. Lay participants without formal training relied on a commonsense index that demonstrated both lower construct and convergent validity.

The formalized index used by FDEs was more comprehensive than the commonsense index used by laypeople. FDEs made more distinctions among the features than did lay participants. FDEs reported that a greater variety of features carried high evidential weight than did lay participants. Lay participants reported consistently high evidential weight for those features they identified, while the evidential weight of features varied more among FDEs.

FDEs made more accurate calls than did lay participants, but FDEs made a greater number of qualified calls, indicating that they afforded different evidential weight to the features they evaluated. Inter-rater reliability among FDEs was higher than that among lay participants. The extent and kind of training, education, and experience was not related to the type and number of features FDEs extracted or the weight they assigned this information, or to the extent to which FDEs outperformed lay participants.

10.11   Signature and handwriting verification systems

Further information regarding the characteristics of forged signatures can be found in the vast body of research associated with the development of signature verification systems (e.g., Plamondon and Lorette 1989; Leclerc and Plamondon 1993; Gupta 2006; Impedevo and Pirlo 2008; Radhika et al. 2008a,b). This research attempts to develop computerized systems that can accurately determine whether a signature is genuine or forged at the point where the signature is being written. The methods are developed both for online as well as offline signatures.

Some computerized systems have also been developed to aid FDEs. Software such as CEDAR-FOX employs distance statistics to determine the authenticity of a questioned signature. The aim of such software is to increase the objectivity of signature and handwriting examinations (Srihari and Leedham 2003). Another system called FLASH-ID is being developed by Gannon Technologies in conjunction with George Mason University. This system is language-independent and has reported significant success in experimental trials (Walch et al. 2009). Other researchers are investigating the possibilities of computer-based forensic handwriting analysis (Franke and Koppen 2001; Franke et al. 2002, 2003; Franke and Rose 2004; Franke and Schomaker 2004).

Signature verification is of great interest to computer scientists both for off-line and on-line systems. There are competitions that are held in which scientists and programmers vie to provide systems that have the highest authentication scores with the fewest errors (Blankers et al. 2009; Liwicki et al. 2010).

10.12   Automation in the forensic examination of handwriting

The USSS and the BKA maintain databases known as the FISH, with the USSS version containing handwriting specimens from a combined 110 000+ writers. To date, no two writers have been found to have the same combination of handwriting characteristics.

At a NIST Measurement Science and Standards in Forensic Handwriting Analysis Conference in June 2013, Dr. Katrin Franke presented "WANDA: A Measurement Tool for Forensic Document Examiners." "She stated that two computer-based forensic handwriting examination systems were operational in Forensic Laboratories, SCRIPT (NIFO/TNO, Netherlands) and FISH (Bundeskriminalamt, Germany). The FISH Database (31 December 1997) had 77 000 investigation cases, 17 500 handwritten products, 32 000 persons, 78 000 identifications of persons, and 86 000 documents. Since 1988 FISH is operating in forensic labs. Handwriting is: classified by shape characteristics, compared with database, presented according to recognized similarities, digitally stored, and managed." Dr. Franke is currently upgrading the FISH system which is now called "WANDA."

The CEDAR, at the State University of New York, continues to conduct studies using computer software to measure handwriting features. In a published study of over 1500 writers (Srihari et al. 2002), the computer system was able to identify the correct writer with a 95% confidence level. Their automated system CEDAR-FOX has been operational for years and narrows down the possibility of writers which is continually being updated. Now the center is developing "iFox" that will assist the FDE in going the last mile (e.g., associate probabilities with their observations).

FLASH ID software is being developed by Gannon Technologies in conjunction with the FBI. This system is reported to be a handwriting identification system that is language-independent (Gantz and Walch 2013).

10.13 Current research

There are several studies in handwriting that are being funded through competitive grant awards from the National Institute of Justice. These are the following:

Frequency Occurrence of Handwriting and Hand-Printing Characteristics—University of Central Florida—Grant No.: 2010-DN-BX-K273. Development of Individual Handwriting Characteristics in 1800 Students: Statistical Analysis and Likelihood Ratios That Emerge over an Extended Period of Time—Minnesota Bureau of Criminal Apprehension—Grant No.: 2010-DN-BX-K212.

Cognitive Human Factors and Forensic Document Examiner Methods and Procedures—Kentucky State University—Grant No.: 2015-DN-BX-K069.

These studies will add empirical data to the field of handwriting examination that should additionally support the foundations of the field.

Currently in the United States, when the FDE makes a subjective judgment as to whether the signature is genuine, disguised, or forged, this judgment is often stated as an opinion as detailed in the "ASTM International Standard E1658-08: Standard Terminology for Expressing the Conclusions of Forensic Document Examiners." This standard is also available as a Scientific Working Group for Document Examiners (SWGDOC) standard and can be accessed at www.swgdoc.org.

The standard provides FDEs with a nine-point scale: (i) Identification (wrote); (ii) Most probably wrote; (iii) Probably wrote; (iv) Indications wrote; (v) Inconclusive; (vi) Indications did not write; (vii) Probably did not write; (viii) Most probably did not write; (ix) Elimination (Did not write).

Some FDEs use the entire scale, while others may use seven, five, or even three points. Other forensic scientists (including FDEs) have criticized the use of the ASTM scale and prefer to express their opinions within the Bayesian logical framework. Further research is needed to determine what the best scale is.

10.14 Conclusion

10.14.1 The public and how law and forensics will be shaped
Some States have no FDEs in their State Crime Laboratories and some have reduced their number. Terrorism cases are on the rise and bank robberies with notes is booming. Identity theft and credit card fraud are out of control. White collar crime, including mortgage fraud in all aspects is barely looked at forensically. The public has limited access to government laboratories for lower-level fraud. Hopefully, these areas will be addressed by the appropriate agencies.

FDEs will continue to conduct examinations as described earlier. Some law enforcement agencies have begun hiring FDEs to handle the large number of cases previously unaddressed. I believe more and more of the local government cases will be handled by private document examiners the way it was in the first half of the 1900s.

10.14.2 Research

As presented, we can see the large amount of research in the FDE area being conducted and followed up upon. Experts will continue to collaborate with academics and researchers to objectively quantify handwriting features through computer software, establish the frequency of specific handwriting and hand printing characteristics in heterogeneous and homogenous population of writers. Studies will be conducted on writing development of elementary schoolchildren to determine when individuality emerges, especially with some schools not teaching cursive handwriting and only teaching students to print. Continuation of the research studies of the neuroscience behind motor control and kinematics of handwriting and hopefully more eye-tracking studies that differentiate experts from laypeople. This should help the designer of automated handwriting identification systems. Future research in handwriting will continue to "push" computer technology until it is capable of human pattern analysis abilities so that variable features can be quantified and frequency of occurrence of specific features can be established. Continue proficiency testing studies to establish error rates in other handwriting examinations, such as disguised writing, limited quantity of writing and foreign-born writing, and statistical confidence levels to the conclusion scale.

10.14.3 Research in other document examinations

Establish statistical methods to forensically differentiate office machine technologies, such as scanners, printers, and copiers. Proficiency testing to establish error rates in QD examinations such as office machines, indented writing, and counterfeit documents.

References

ABFDE n.d. [Internet]. Houston: American Board of Forensic Document Examiners, Background, Functions and Purposes of the ABFDE (28 June 2011). http://www.abfde.org/htdocs/AboutABFDE/BackgroundFunctionsPurposes.pdf

ASTM Standard E444 (2009, 2009). *Standard Guide for Scope of Work of Forensic Document Examiners*. West Conshohocken, PA: ASTM International.

Beacom, M.S. (1960). A statistical study of handwritings by twins and other persons of multiple births. *Journal of Forensic Sciences* 5: 121–131.

Blankers, V., van den Heuvel, E., Franke, K., and Vuurpijl, L. (2009). The ICDAR 2009 signature verification competition. *Proceedings of the 10th International Conference on Document Analysis and Recognition*, Barcelona, Spain.

Boot, D. (1998). An investigation into the degree of similarity in the handwriting of identical and fraternal twins in New Zealand. *Journal of the American Society of Questioned Document Examiners* 1: 70–81.

Bradford, R.R. and Bradford, R. (1992). *Introduction to Handwriting Examination and Identification*. Chicago: Nelson-Hall.

Caligiuri, M., Mohammed, L., Found, B., and Rogers, D. (2012). Nonadherence to the isochrony principle in forged signatures. *Forensic Science International* 223 (1–3): 228–232.

Caligiuri, M., Kim, C., and Landy, K. (2014). Kinematics of signature writing in healthy aging. *Journal of Forensic Sciences* 59 (4): 1020–1024.

Chabot, C. and Twisleton, E.T.B. (1871). *The Handwriting of Junius, Professionally Investigated by Mr. Charles Chabot, Expert*[Internet]. London: J Murray.

Coupland, V. (2004). A critical evaluation of two methods of signature analysis. *Science and Justice* 44 (2): 65–71.

Crown, D. (1989). Questioned document examination. In: *Forensic Sciences Law/Science Civil/Criminal*, vol. 3 (ed. C.H. Wecht). New York: Matthew Bender & Co, Inc.; 39:9.

Durina, M. and Caligiuri, M.P. (2009). The determination of authorship from a homogenous group of writers. *Journal of the American Society of Forensic Document Examiners* 12: 77–90.

Dyer, A., Found, B., and Rogers, D. (2008). An insight into forensic document examiner expertise for discriminating between forged and disguised signatures. *Journal of Forensic Sciences* 53 (5): 1154–1159.

Franke, K. (2009). Analysis of authentic signatures and forgeries. *Computational Forensics. Third International Workshop Proceedings, IWCF*, The Hague, The Netherlands (13–14 August).

Franke, K. and Koppen, M. (2001). A computer-based system to support forensic studies on handwritten documents. *International Journal on Document Analysis and Recognition* 3 (4): 218–231.

Franke, K. & Rose, S. (2004). Ink-deposition model: the relation of writing and ink deposition processes. *Proceedings of the 9th International Workshop on Frontiers in Handwriting Recognition (IWFHR)*, Tokyo, Japan: 173–178.

Franke, K. and Schomaker, L. (2004). Robotic writing trace synthesis and its application in the study of signature line quality. *Journal of Forensic Document Examination* 16: 119–146.

Franke, K., Zhang, Y., and Köppen, M. (2002). Static signature verification employing a Kosko–Neuro–Fuzzy approach. In: *Advances in Soft Computing – AFSS 2002, LNAI 2275* (ed. N.R. Pal and M. Sugeno), 185–190. Springer Verlag.

Franke, K., Schomaker, L., Veenhuis, C. et al. (2003). WANDA: a generic framework applied in forensic handwriting analysis and writer identification, design and application of hybrid intelligent systems. In: *Proceedings of the 3rd International Conference on Hybrid Intelligent Systems (HIS03)* (ed. A. Abraham, M. Köppen and K. Franke), 927–938. Amsterdam, The Netherlands: IOS Press.

Gamble, D.J. (1980). The handwriting of identical twins. *Canadian Society of Forensic Journal* 13: 11–30.

Gantz, D. and Walch, M. (2013). *FLASH ID Handwriting Derived Biometric Analysis Software. NIST Measurement Science and Standards in Forensic Handwriting Analysis Conference*, Washington, DC.

van Gemmert, A. and van Galen, G. (1996). Dynamical features of mimicking another person's writing and signature. In: *Handwriting and Drawing Research: Basic and Applied Issues* (ed. M.L. Simner, C.G. Leedham and A.J.W.M. Thomassen), 459–471. Amsterdam: IOP Press.

van Galen, G. (1984). Structural complexity of motor patterns: A study on reaction times of handwritten letters. *Psychological Research* 46 (1–2): 49–57.

van Gemmert, A., van Galen, G., Hardy, H., and Thomassen, A. (1996). Dynamical features of disguised handwriting. *Proceedings of the Fifth European Conference for Police and Government Handwriting Experts*, The Hague, The Netherlands.

Gupta, G. (2006). *The State of the Art in On-line Handwritten Signature Verification*. Melbourne: Monash University.

Hilton, O. (1979). History of questioned document examination in the United States. *Journal of Forensic Sciences* 24 (4): 890–897.

Hilton, O. (1993). *Scientific Examination of Questioned Documents*. Boca Raton, FL: CRC Press.

Huber, R.A. and Headrick, A.M. (1999). *Handwriting Identification Facts & Fundamentals*, 3–8. New York: CRC Press.

Impedevo, D. and Pirlo, G. (2008). Automatic signature verification: the state of the art. *IEEE Transactions on Systems, Man, and Cybernetics, Part C: Applications and Reviews* 38 (5): 609–635.

Kam, M. and Lin, E. (2003). Writer identification using hand-printed and non-hand-printed questioned documents. *Journal of Forensic Sciences* 48: 1391–1395.

Kam, M., Wetstein, J., and Corm, R. (1994, 1994). Proficiency of professional document examiners in writer identification. *Journal of Forensic Sciences* 39: 5–14.

Kam, M., Fielding, G., and Conn, R. (1997). Writer identification by professional document examiners. *Journal of Forensic Sciences* 42: 778–786.

Kam, M., Gummadidala, K., Fielding, G., and Conn, R. (2001, 2001). Signature authentication by forensic document examiners. *Journal of Forensic Sciences* 46: 884–888.

Kelly, J.S. and Lindblom, B.S. (2006). *Scientific Examination of Questioned Documents*, 2e. Boca Raton, FL: CRC Press.

Leclerc, F. and Plamondon, R. (1993). Automatic signature verification: the state of the art 1989–1993. *International Journal of Pattern Recognition and Artificial Intelligence* 8 (3): 644–660.

Levinson, J. (2001). *Questioned Documents, A Lawyer's Handbook*, 1–7. San Diego: Academic Press.

Liwicki, M., van den Heuvel, E., Found, B., and Malik, M. (2010). Forensic signature verification competition: detection of simulated and disguised signatures. *Proceedings of the 12th International Conference on Frontiers on Handwriting Recognition*, Kolkata, India.

Louisiana Supreme Court (1854). *Reports of Cases Argued and Determined by the Supreme Court of Louisiana, Volume 7, for the Year 1852*, 565–566. New Orleans: T Rea.

McAlexander, T.V., Beck, J., and Dick, R. (1991). The standardization of handwriting opinion terminology. *Journal of Forensic Sciences* 36 (2): 313.

Merlino, M., Freeman, T., Dahir, V., et al. (2014). Validity, Reliability, Accuracy, and Bias in Forensic Signature Identification. *Final Tech. Rep. NIJ Award Number 2010-DN-BX-K271*.

Moenssens, A. and Inbau, F. (1978). *Scientific Evidence in Civil and Criminal Cases*. Mineola, NY: Foundation Press, Inc.

Mohammed, L., Found, B., Caligiuri, M., and Rogers, D. (2011). The dynamic character of disguise behavior for text-based, mixed, and stylized signatures. *Journal of Forensic Sciences* 56 (S1): S136–S141.

Mohammed, L., Found, B., Caligiuri, M., and Rogers, D. (2015). Dynamic characteristics of signatures: effects of writer style on genuine and simulated signatures. *Journal of Forensic Sciences* 60 (1): 89–94.

Osborn, A.S. (1929). *Questioned Documents*, 2e. Albany, NY: Boyd Printing Company.

Albert S. Osborn (1992) ASQDE [Internet]: Long Beach, CA: American Society of Questioned Document Examiners; c1997-2011. http://www.asqde.org/about/presidents/osborn_as.html

Osborn, A.S. (1922). *The Problem of Proof*, 2e. Albany, NY/Newark, NJ: Essex Press.

Plamondon, R. and Lorette, G. (1989). Automatic signature verification and writer identification – the state of the art. *Pattern Recognition* 22: 107–131.

Radhika, K., Venkatesha, M., and Sekhar, G. (2008a). Handwritten signature verification methods. *Proceedings of the World Academy of Science, Engineering and Technology* 36: 884–890.

Radhika, K., Venkatesha, M., and Sekhar, G. (2008b). Pattern recognition techniques in off-line hand written signature verification – a survey. *Proceedings of the World Academy of Science, Engineering and Technology* 36: 905–911.

Riordan, W.M., Gustafson, J.A., Fitzgerald, M.P., and Lewis, J.A. (2012). Forensic document examination. In: *Forensic Science: Current Issues, Future Directions* (ed. D.H. Ubelaker), 224–251. West Sussex: Wiley Blackwell.

Robertson, E.W. (1991). *Fundamentals of Document Examination*. Chicago: Nelson-Hall.

Sita, J., Found, B., and Rogers, D. (2002). Forensic handwriting examiners' expertise for signature comparison. *Journal of Forensic Sciences* 47: 1117–1124.

Srihari, S., Huang, C., and Srinivasan, H. (2008). On the discriminability of the handwriting of twins. *Journal of Forensic Sciences* 53 (2): 431–446.

Srihari, S. and Leedham, G. (2003). A survey of computer methods in forensic document examination. In: *Proceedings of the 11th Conference of the International Graphonomics Society* (ed. H.L. Teulings and A.W.A. van Gemmert). Scottsdale, Arizona. www.graphonomics.org..

Srihari, S.N., Cha, S.H., Arora, H., and Lee, S. (2002). The individuality of handwriting. *Journal of Forensic Sciences* 47 (4): 856–872.

SWGDOC n.d. [Internet]. Scientific Working Group for Forensic Document Examination [updated 2011 Nov 15]. About SWGDOC; [updated 2011 Sep 22]. http://www.swgdoc.org/about_us.htm.

The Origin of the ASQDE n.d. [Internet]: Long Beach, CA: American Society of Questioned Document Examiners; c1997-2011. www.asqde.org/about/history.html

Walch, M., Gantz, D., Miller, J., and Buscaglia, J. (2009). Evaluation of the language-independent process in the FLASH ID System for handwriting identification. Presented at the American Academy of Forensic Sciences Conference, Denver, Colorado.

Further readings

Aitken, C., Berger, C., Buckleton, J. et al. (2011). Expressing evaluative opinions – a position statement. *Science and Justice* 51 (1): 1–2.

American Board of Forensic Document Examiners (ABFDE) [Internet] 2014. http://www.abfde.org.

Berger, C., Buckleton, J., Champod, C. et al. (2011). Evidence evaluation: a response to the court of appeal judgment in R v T. *Science and Justice* 51 (2): 43–49.

Caligiuri, M. and Mohammed, L. (2012). *The Neuroscience of Handwriting: Applications for Forensic Document Examination.* Boca Raton, FL: Taylor & Francis. [Suggested by speaker John Sang].

Ellen, D. (2006). *Scientific Examination of Documents: Methods and Techniques,* 3e. Boca Raton, FL: CRC Press.

Ellen Schuetnzer's Database (FDE Testimony List) lists more than 3,200 FDE testimonies since 1993. It contains cases in which a judge or hearing officer has allowed a document examiner to testify to his/her findings. This list contains cases from Daubert (1993) to present. The Forensic Document Examiner Testimony List, Ellen M. Schuetzner, BA, presented at AAFS meeting 2015.

ENFSI (n.d.) [Internet]. The Hague: European Network of Forensic Science Institutes; c1999–2009. European Document

Evett, I. (1998). Handwriting, probability, and the nature of the science. Presentation at the Joint Meeting of the European Conferences for Police and Government Handwriting Experts, Tulliallan, Scotland.

Evett, I., Jackson, G., Lambert, J., and McCrossan, S. (2000). The impact of the principles of evidence interpretation on the structure and content of statements. *Science and Justice* 40 (4): 233–239.

Franke, K. (2013). WANDA: *A Measurement Tool for Forensic Document Examiners. NIST Measurement Science and Standards in Forensic Handwriting Analysis Conference,* Washington, DC.

Franke, K. and Grube, G. (1998). The automatic extraction of pseudodynamic information from static images of handwriting based on marked gray value segmentation. *Journal of Forensic Document Examination* 11: 17–38.

Harris, J.J. (1998). A tribute to Ordway Hilton. *ABFDE News* 9 (3): pp. 1, 17.

Harrison, W.R. (1958). *Suspect Documents, Their Scientific Examination.* New York, NY: Praeger.

Kam, M., Fielding, G., and Conn, R. (1998). Effects of monetary incentives on performance of nonprofessionals in document examination proficiency tests. *Journal of Forensic Sciences* 43: 1000–1004.

Koller, N., Kai, N., Rieb, M., and Sadorf, E. (2004). *Probability Conclusions in Expert Opinions on Handwriting. Substantiation and Standardization of Probability Statements in Expert Opinions.* Munchen: Wolters Kluwer Deutschland GmbH.

Lewis, J. (2014). *Forensic Document Examination: Fundamentals and Current Trends.* Oxford: Academic Press.

Moenssens, A., Henderson, C., and Portwood, S.G. (2007). *Scientific Evidence in Civil and Criminal Cases.* New York, NY: Foundation Press.

Morris, R.N. (2000). *Forensic Handwriting Identification: Fundamental Concepts and Principles.* London: Academic Press.

Scientific Working Group for Forensic Document Examination [Internet]. 2012. http://www.swgdoc.org

Singer, K. (2006). The Daubert era. In: *Scientific Examination of Questioned Documents* (ed. S. Kelly and B.S. Lindblom), 37–42. Boca Raton: CRC Taylor & Francis.

Srihari, S. (2013). *Role of Automation in the Forensic Examination of Handwritten Items. NIST Measurement Science and Standards in Forensic Handwriting Analysis Conference*, Washington, DC.

Measurement science and standards in forensic handwriting analysis – U.S. Commerce Department's National Institute of Standards and Technology (NIST) Symposium, June 2013 presentations

Neuroscience Behind the Motor Control and Motor Equivalence of the Handwriting Function – Dr. Michael Caligiuri, Professor, University of California – San Diego.

Handwriting Stroke Kinematics – Linton Mohammed, PhD, D-ABFDE, Forensic Document Examiner, Forensic Science Consultants, Inc.

Cognitive Theoretical Perspectives in Studies of Forensic Document Examination including "What Examiners Look At" (i.e., Eye-tracking) – Dr. Mara Merlino, Assistant Professor of Psychology, Kentucky State University.

The Forensic Language-Independent Analysis System for Handwriting Identification (FLASH ID) – Mark Walch, President CEO, Gannon Technologies Group and Dr. Don Gantz, Statistician, George Mason University.

Forensic Information System for Handwriting (FISH) – Kathleen Storer, Forensic Document Examiner, United States Secret Service.

WANDA: A Measurement Tool for Forensic Document Examiners – Dr. Katrin Franke, Professor of Computer Science and Director of the Digital Forensics and Cybercrime Investigation Laboratory at Gjøvik University College.

Scale Invariant Feature Transform (SIFT) – Dr. Jeff Woodard, Researcher, Mitre.

D-Scribe – Matthias Schulte-Austum, Siemens AG, Senior Software Development Engineer and Siemens Key Expert Pattern Recognition.

CEDAR FOX and iFOX – Dr. Sargur Srihari, PhD, Distinguished Professor, Department of Computer Science and Engineering, and Director of the Center of Excellence for Document Analysis and Recognition, State University of New York (SUNY), Buffalo, NY.

CHAPTER 11

Past perspectives and future directions in forensic toxicology

Barry K. Logan[1] F-ABFT

Chief Scientist, NMS Labs
Center for Forensic Science Research and Education (CFSRE) at the Fredric Rieders Family Foundation, Willow Grove, PA, USA

11.1 Our history

Forensic toxicology is the science of drugs and poisons and the medicolegal consequences of their use. This encompasses applications in assisting with determination of the role of toxic substances in medicolegal death investigations and assignment of cause and manner of death; identifying substances that might cause impairment in a person's cognitive or psychomotor skills, especially as it relates to driving or the operation of machinery; and finally, testing for the presence of drugs in a variety of regulated environments such as transportation, the workplace, or in sports. There are two major domains to forensic toxicology—analytical toxicology and interpretive toxicology. The former is today a highly technology-driven laboratory-based science requiring in depth knowledge of chemistry and physics, and the latter, a complex expert domain requiring knowledge of pharmacology, behavioral psychology, biochemistry, anatomy and physiology, and mammalian systems toxicology. Forensic toxicology is a strong science-based discipline within forensic science, however, like all areas of science, it faces opportunities and challenges as it continues to grow and mature.

---

[1]The author is employed by a commercial forensic toxicology reference laboratory and makes reference in the article to the services offered by private reference laboratories.

The Future of Forensic Science, First Edition. Edited by Daniel A. Martell.
© 2019 John Wiley & Sons Ltd. Published 2019 by John Wiley & Sons Ltd.

Although knowledge of the therapeutic and toxic effects of plant, animal, and mineral poisons goes back to ancient history, our ability to test for them is relatively new. The derivation of chemical structures and pharmacological mechanisms from advances in chemistry and pharmacology have formed the basis of today's practice of forensic toxicology.

Most people in the field point to the establishment of Alexander O. Gettler's laboratory at the Office of the Medical Examiner in New York City in 1918 as the beginning of forensic toxicology in the United States. For some historical context, the structure of morphine was not elucidated until 1925, by Sir Robert Robinson; oxycodone and hydrocodone, the first semisynthetic opioids were not invented until the 1920s, and most "pharmaceuticals" of the time were simply plant extracts. Tests for the presence of drugs in toxicological tissues were performed using extractions of liver tissue or gastric contents (where drugs and toxins are most concentrated) and their characterization using crystal tests and color tests, melting point determination, and titration. It is fascinating to reflect on the innovative yet simple and sense-based processes these early toxicologists used to detect potentially toxic substances in their investigations—for example, smelling for the presence of the odor of almonds to detect cyanide poisoning, deposition of a metallic mirror on a glass surface by liberation of arsenic or thallium from tissue samples.

Many toxicologists received their training in Gettler's laboratory and took that learning to establish forensic toxicology laboratories at major medical examiners offices and academic institutions around the United States. Major milestones in the advancement of analytical capabilities included the introduction of the Beckman UV Spectrophotometer in 1941, which enabled more accurate quantitative analysis for drugs such as salicylates, barbiturates, and acetaminophen, and in 1967, the introduction of the Perkin Elmer GC-900 gas chromatograph for blood alcohol testing, replacing older, labor-intensive but still accurate titrimetric methods with more stable, faster approaches. Other instrument vendors improved the technology, and costs declined making instrumentation more accessible. The HP 5990 benchtop gas chromatograph mass spectrometer was introduced by Hewlett Packard in 1976. In 1979, fused silica capillary columns were introduced by HP, improving sensitivity and reducing analysis times. Solid phase extraction columns were introduced in the 1980s, and affordable benchtop Liquid Chromatography–Mass Spectrometry (LCMS) systems became available in the early 2000s, improving sensitivity yet again, and enabling detection of more challenging and more potent drugs. Today, we are seeing the impact of the introduction of high-resolution mass spectrometry (HRMS), including time of flight (TOF) and quadrupole time of flight (QTOF) approaches, a key advancement that will change the face of forensic toxicology one more time.

As noted earlier, there is more to forensic toxicology than the ability to detect the presence of poisons, drugs, or toxins. Once the agents have been detected, identified, and measured, the toxicologists' greater challenge is in their interpretation. Early tools for this included the compilation of compendia of drug concentrations into therapeutic, toxic, and fatal ranges. A staple of toxicological interpretation through the 1990s was tables produced by Dr. Charles Winek, of the Allegheny County Medical Examiners Office and by Dr. Donald Uges in the Netherlands, for The International Association of Forensic Toxicologists (TIAFT). Toxicologists quickly learned, however, that a one-size-fits-all approach to interpretation didn't work, as there was so much overlap between concentrations in the different categories. Drs. Randall Baselt and Robert Cravey began the immense task of compiling and summarizing reports, studies and case series from the medical and scientific literature into a collection of monographs that became and remain today, the most authoritative and widely relied upon textbook in the field, *Disposition of Toxic Drugs and Chemicals in Man*. This became the "Bible" of forensic toxicology and remains a key text today, currently in its 11th edition.

In the human performance arena, alcohol had been the most studied drug, most notably with early work by the Swedish scientist Dr. Erik Widmark in the 1930s. Alcohol testing has become routine and is almost universally performed by headspace gas chromatography with flame ionization detection. Dr. Robert Borkenstein invented the Breathalyzer in 1956, and he began a program at Indiana University to train police officers and forensic scientists in program implementation, the pharmacology and effects of alcohol on driving and skills involved in courtroom testimony. That program continues today at IU and has trained over 5000 individuals from around the world.

A key discovery made in the 1980s by members of the profession concerned the dynamic nature of the postmortem condition. Richard Prouty and Drs. Bill Anderson, Graham Jones, and others began reporting on the phenomenon of postmortem redistribution (PMR) of drugs, and the realization that many factors contributed to differences in concentration of drugs between sites and tissue types. In addition, the fact that drug concentrations can change during the postmortem interval, where drugs are released from tissue into the fluids, and fluids can continue to move after death as a result of settling and putrefactive changes. This generated a greater recognition of the importance of the consideration of the whole case—the investigative, autopsy and toxicological findings when assigning a cause of death.

In addition to the growth from the development of technology, and greater insight into the mechanisms of toxicity and the dynamic nature of postmortem change, the field of forensic science and the discipline of forensic toxicology began to professionalize. The American Academy of Forensic Sciences (AAFS) was formed in 1948, and toxicology was one of the first sections recognized by the new organization. In 1975, with support from the AAFS, the American Board of Forensic Toxicology (ABFT) was formed with the goal of establishing minimum standards and qualifications for practitioners of forensic toxicology. In 1997, ABFT also began to provide accreditation of laboratories, based on guidelines developed by the joint AAFS/Society of Forensic Toxicologists (SOFT) Laboratory Guidelines Committee. These steps of establishing voluntary certification criteria for individuals, and accreditation criteria for laboratories, improved the quality and reliability of forensic toxicology testing and interpretation, and paved the way for some of the other key developments in the field. One of these was the establishment in 2009 of the Scientific Working Group for Toxicology (SWGTOX) to further develop and continuously improve quality standards. Those activities later transitioned to the National Institute for Standards and Technology's (NIST's) Organization of Scientific Area Committees (OSAC) in Forensic Science (discussed later in section 11.3.2), which is now taking the process of standards development to the next level through a public and transparent consensus-based standards development process.

Another major driver for change and process improvement in the forensic sciences was the issuance of the report in 2009 by the National Academies of Sciences' on "Strengthening Forensic Science in the United States—A Path Forward." Forensic toxicology and drug chemistry fared quite well in that review, with the Academies reporting that these sciences were derived from well-understood principles in basic research, and that the methods and technologies had gone through the process of validation and peer review, and withstood that scrutiny. General concerns concerning any quantitative science raised by the Academies, certainly apply to forensic toxicology measurements, including understanding error rates, measurement uncertainty, clarity of reporting, and issues related to the need for ongoing research, and the training of the next generation of forensic scientists, are issues this discipline has begun to address.

11.2   Reflections on factors affecting our future direction

Reflecting on the history of our profession in forensic toxicology, the last 30 years have been extremely exciting, and ever-changing. In the early 2000s, the practice had become much improved. There is more emphasis on quality and quality control, better documentation of our work, the sensitivity of the instrumentation was sufficient for the detection of forensically significant quantities of most drugs and toxins, we had resources to aid with interpretation, and were more conservative in our approach, and we were working more closely with medical examiners and pathologists as part of a team in the determination of cause of death. Medical examiners and pathologists, for the most part, knew to collect peripheral blood for testing which helped with the interpretation of results. The stability and robustness of the testing processes and technology, and the availability of affordable, fit-for-purpose equipment had made the analytical component of the field more straightforward.

Just as the forensic toxicology community had recognized and embraced the value of standardization and accreditation, so too had the forensic pathology and medical examiner community. In 1975, the National Association of Medical Examiners (NAME) had developed an accreditation process and was developing an autopsy standards document, which emphasized the importance of forensic toxicology as part of a comprehensive death investigation. This has led to better utilization of toxicology resources by pathologists and medical examiners. Likewise, a similar process has been taking place with the development of the American Board of Medicolegal Death Investigation (ABMDI) that reinforces the importance of forensic toxicology and has further contributed to the demand for testing.

There was a growing appreciation in the late 1990s and early 2000s of the significant involvement of drugs in impairment of the cognitive and psychomotor skills needed for safe driving. Previously that focus had been on alcohol, which was very well understood in terms of its pharmacokinetics, effects, and analysis. The implementation of drug testing in the workplace in the 1990s had raised awareness of the extent of drug use in society, and inevitably among some individuals in safety sensitive jobs. More presentations at professional meetings and publications began to document drugs associated with impairment in drivers, rates of testing increased, and toxicologists began to train and prepare themselves for testimony. In 2002, the Borkenstein Drug Course was started at Indiana University to complement the alcohol course. A synergy developed between toxicologists and the Drug Recognition and Evaluation (DRE) program developed by the National Highway Traffic Safety Administration (NHTSA), where the objective effects of drug impairment are documented onsite by observation, and the toxicological information from a test of the subjects blood, urine, and eventually oral fluid, establishes the nexus between the observed effects, and the subject's drug ingestion. The program has become widely adopted throughout the United States, and consequently requests for drug testing in impaired driving cases began to increase.

The laboratory accreditation program established by ABFT in 1996, and the inclusion of toxicology as a discipline in the American Society of Crime Laboratory Directors—Laboratory Accreditation Board (ASCLD-LAB) inspections, while improving quality and documentation of testing, created significant additional demands on laboratories to hire staff related to managing all the requirements to attain and support accreditation, and to maintain the documentation of instrument maintenance, method validation, quality control, personnel training, traceability, uncertainty of measurement, and many other requirements needed to demonstrate compliance with the accreditation criteria.

This confluence of greater demand for toxicological testing in human performance and postmortem toxicology and the additional resources needed to support and maintain compliance with accreditation made toxicological testing more expensive, and unfortunately in the government sector, many laboratories were not provided with the resources needed to do both. Backlogs began to build, and in 2019 in many jurisdictions, these still persist.

An additional challenge impacting toxicology practice today arrived in the late 2000s with the advent of the novel psychoactive substances (NPS) explosion, and later, starting in 2015, the opioids crisis.

The NPS era began in about 2008 with the advent of synthetic cannabinoid agents in Europe. These were substances markedly different in structure and functional group chemistry from delta-9-tetrahydrocannabinol (THC)—the active component in marijuana. Nevertheless, these synthetic cannabinoids (dubbed "Designer Drugs" at the time) had significant receptor binding at the CB1 receptor which is responsible for the well-known effect profile of marijuana and produced marijuana-like effects. The synthetic cannabinoids were followed by a series of cathinone-derived, β-keto amphetamine stimulants, or pyrovalerone-class hallucinogens, entactogens, and entheogens, the so-called "Bath Salts" compounds. Novel opioids and benzodiazepines followed in 2014 and 2015. The development and proliferation of fentanyl analogs and other novel mu receptor agonists represents one of the most diverse categories of new drugs, and their high potency and toxicity made their detection in medicolegal death investigation casework critical.

The NPS era has created five major challenges for forensic toxicologists, which persist today in dealing with each successive wave of new substances and each new class of NPS.

The first challenge is the change in model from an environment where new analytes came along infrequently and of which most were novel therapeutic drugs that had been well studied and characterized by the pharmaceutical industry and academic researchers before their launch. In the NPS arena, new substances with both quite divergent chemistries, and closely related analogs and isomers within each new chemical class of substances is the norm. The substances have rarely been studied in animal models or human trials, little is known about their potency or toxicity, or their metabolism. Preparing to test, identify, and interpret NPS findings in toxicological casework has strained laboratories ability to keep their scope of testing up to date, and to frequently and rapidly validate new or updated methods in an accreditation-compliant manner.

Many legacy techniques, commonplace in toxicology laboratories— immunoassay, and gas chromatography–mass spectrometry (GCMS), are not sufficiently sensitive to detect many of these novel potent drugs and their metabolites. GCMS does not have sufficient mass resolution to tease apart the structural detail of the emerging drugs. So the second challenge toxicology faces is in acquiring and mastering new screening technologies with the necessary sensitivity and resolving power to both identify novel substances that are often not in the libraries and databases. This by and large means the use of HRMS on TOF and QTOF platforms. The chemical problem-solving skills required in recognizing something in analytical data that is out-of-the-ordinary, and performing the necessary follow-up work to identify it, are skills that we have not had to rely on when testing menus were a lot more stable, and true unknowns or novel drugs came along a lot less frequently. Obtaining the instrumentation is itself costly (HRMS platforms cost from \$650 000 to \$800 000), but the associated costs of hiring more experienced analysts to develop and validate the tests, training other analysts in the operation of the technology, and the costs of reviewing and analyzing the more complex data coming from these instruments are hidden costs that are often overlooked. This can result in expensive potentially powerful instrumentation arriving in the laboratory, but having no resource to put it into practice.

Third, current standards of forensic practice require that results are verified by comparison to a certified standard reference material (SRM). Since many of these substances are very new, frequently commercial vendors do not have available SRM's at the time of their first discovery, delaying method development and validation. When

SRM's are not commercially available, custom synthesis can be very costly (several thousand dollars per compound) and time-consuming, making it a poor option. Some of the SRM suppliers are outside of the United States, and there can be delays in importation, licensing, and delivery of these materials. This is more of a problem in other countries than in the United States, but is still a significant consideration.

Fourth, once the laboratory has the equipment, has trained its staff to operate it, SRM's have been ordered and acquired, and the method is developed, validated, and signed-off, the samples have to be tested, on top of the already heavy demands for testing. While a few NPS proliferate widely and become quite prevalent most of them do not, so laboratories may have to develop, validate, and run multiple methods, each with very few samples, which is a very inefficient and costly approach.

Finally, once the results for these novel substances have been generated, what do they mean? With traditional drugs of abuse and therapeutics that have been around for a long time, or that were thoroughly studied in supervised trials and those results published in the peer-reviewed literature, there are readily accessible reference data to compare results to. With NPS, since prevalence is low compared to say heroin or cocaine, there are few case reports or case series in the literature with which to compare the latest case. This means that there is a period of time during which data are collected, but often are not shared, or the cases not published or presented in a timely manner, leaving the user of the report—the investigator, coroner, medical examiner or prosecutor, with a limited basis on which to interpret the result or to utilize it. Finding better ways to more rapidly share this data with stakeholder groups is one of the biggest opportunities for development and advancement in forensic toxicology as discussed later.

11.3   Facing forward

From this vantage point in 2018, with the learnings identified above there are clear opportunities and challenges for the discipline of forensic toxicology moving forward, to maximize the value of the services and data that toxicology labs are capable of providing.

11.3.1   Laboratory resources and the role of the Federal Government

Forensic toxicology laboratories can offer so much more today in terms of scope of analysis, sensitivity than in the past. However, the year-over-year increase in opioid-related deaths (many of them novel opioids), and NPS in impaired driving casework, are all contributing in increases in submission volumes to toxicology labs. Labs have understandably turned to the deep pockets of the Federal Government through organizations like the Consortium of Forensic Science Organizations (CFSO), but ultimately, it is the states for whom the testing is mostly done, who need to bear the primary burden of supporting their own laboratories at appropriate levels. Federal funds are notoriously ephemeral and unpredictable, and local laboratories cannot rely on the vagaries of the Federal Budget, and its changing priorities to support this key local public health and public safety function. Organizations like the National Institute of Justice (NIJ) have done highly commendable work in supporting specific priorities such as DNA kit backlog reduction, and can legitimately support training initiatives, new technology assessment, and encourage research to improve testing and detection capabilities. Federal funds are also key for one-time emergencies, such as helping state and local laboratories with funds for backlog elimination in various disciplines including toxicology, but unless the local agencies and governments step up and fund the ongoing costs of providing this crucial public health/public safety service, we run the risk of never getting out from under current backlogs. Through programs like the NIJ Research Fellowship program, NIJ is helping create the forensic toxicology leaders of tomorrow—a role the importance of which cannot be overstated, and which is discussed later.

11.3.2   Standards development and harmonization of best practices

Probably the most significant contribution of the Federal Government has been in the establishment of the OSAC within the National Institute for Standards and Technology (NIST) at the Department of Commerce. NIST is the pre-eminent scientific research organization within the Federal Government in the area of measurement science and standardization, and its leadership in the establishment of a multidisciplinary, intergovernmental, public/private, stakeholder based initiative to improve quality within the practice of forensic science is one of the greatest developments in the field in the modern era. Forensic toxicology as a discipline has a long history of supporting and encouraging continuous quality improvement in the field. Prior efforts in forensic toxicology at creating best practices recommendations and consensus documents were laudable; specifically the leadership of ABFT, and the SOFT/AAFS Laboratory Guidelines Committee, which led to the work done by SWGTOX, and created an environment and culture that emphasizes quality and the need for more uniformity in testing practices. The OSAC toxicology subcommittee has made great strides in converting those guidelines into true standards through the OSAC's open and transparent consensus-based process. The process with its diversity of input (practitioners, researchers, instrument vendors and standards suppliers; state, local, federal, academic and private practitioners; geographic diversity; and larger and smaller organizations) helps ensure that all practitioner stakeholder groups have a voice. The quality, legal, and human factors review of proposed standards documents, open periods for public comment, and accountability for addressing that comment, create the best forum our field has for creating robust, forensically defensible approaches that meet the quality and legal standards of the courts.

While there is frustration concerning the time it is taking to develop and adopt these standards, this is a complex process, dependent on donated time of the professionals involved and their agencies, on a volunteer basis. The brilliance of the concept of the OSAC, however, is its ability to get buy-in for voluntary adoption of the standards that are ultimately adopted and encourage their incorporation into accreditation requirements. This process will make the practice of our science stronger, reduce the risk of errors, help ensure admissibility of forensic toxicology evidence in court, and improve the weight it is given by the triers-of-fact.

11.3.3   Technology

For the majority of analyses for routine therapeutic and abused drugs, many of the tried and tested techniques are well validated, peer-reviewed, and trusted, and are in widespread use throughout the field. Liquid chromatography/tandem mass spectroscopy (LCMSMS) has seen widespread adoption in recent years and has improved sensitivity for those substances not amenable to GCMS, as well as improving laboratory efficiency. In order to screen for the most challenging NPS compounds however, laboratories will be forced to adopt more nontargeted screening approaches such as those offered by HRMS screening. HRMS allows for greater sensitivity than the GCMS nontargeted approach it is replacing, and coupled to liquid chromatography systems allows for testing without derivatization, with shorter run times, and with less sample preparation. Crucially, nontargeted data acquisition in HRMS allows for archiving electronic data files that can be retrospectively reprocessed and data-mined for novel compounds once we become aware of their existence, without having to store and preserve the sample itself, then retrieve and rescreen it. Confirmatory analysis for the ever-expanding universe of novel substances, many with low prevalence, however suggests that for confirmation of low-frequency, high-complexity confirmation tests, some consolidation of that work into reference laboratories in regional, academic, government, or private centers of excellence will be necessary. This will avoid the very high cost and disruption caused to laboratories without the analytical capacity or the resources for continuous, rapid, method development and validation.

The emerging model is one in which most laboratories will need to upgrade their screening capabilities with HRMS, and focus on confirmation of frequently encountered analytes by GCMS and LCMSMS. For more esoteric and ephemeral analytes, there will be more reliance on reference laboratories for that confirmatory testing. These upgrades to HRMS will be expensive, and this technology transition is a good example of a scenario that warrants an increase in both state and federal funding. Training in particular is an area where government agencies and professional organizations will need to collaborate. The increase in complexity and cost of instrumentation for screening will likely be beyond the reach of many smaller laboratories that cannot afford the expensive technology upgrades, or with the resources to dedicate for accreditation, research, development, and validation.

11.3.4 Training, research, and interdisciplinary collaboration

There has been a proliferation of master's level forensic science programs over the last 15 years, and these have produced many strong scientists who are part of the next generation of leaders in the field. Including practitioners in graduate training programs is critical to the success and relevance of the course materials, and how to put them into practice. These professionals also give the students a realistic idea of what working in the profession entails, in contrast to what is seen in the media. The introduction of Professional Science Masters (PSM) programs in specific disciplines including forensic toxicology, is introducing students to principles of management and leadership, which further enriches our field. Currently, lacking however is more diverse choices for PhD programs with forensic science-based projects closely related to the research needs of the field. Closer cooperation between practicing laboratories and academic programs should also be encouraged as this will help inform the choice of research projects taken on by the graduate students.

Scientists, of course, always believe that "more research is needed," and forensic toxicologists are no different. The complexity of HRMS and LCMSMS platforms that can be operated in multiple different data acquisition modes, will open additional doors to boost sensitivity, scope of testing, and speed of analysis. Programs that encourage interdisciplinary research, for example, between drug chemists and toxicologists will be key, since the rapidly changing drug market has shown that the model of working within silos, that worked when the drug landscape was more stable, no longer works today. Drug chemists often have insight into the appearance of new substances on the market, and sharing that information with their toxicology colleagues will help them be better equipped to recognize these new substances when they appear in fatalities. Likewise, data from death investigation toxicology cases may help provide intelligence to investigators in jurisdictions where novel substances have caused or contributed to deaths, establishing an association between cutting agents or precursors with new substances, and their geographic distribution, to provide insight to where a particular batch of drug may be being distributed.

More research is needed in the area of interpretive toxicology for all substances, in drug interactions, PMR, and genetic differences in drug metabolism. This is especially true with respect to NPS. Early identification of novel substances in the drug market can give researchers a head-start on establishing through receptor binding studies, *in vitro* metabolomics studies, and where needed animal studies of functional effect, better insight into the potency and toxicity of the new substances and an early assessment of their harm. Collecting this information quickly also helps with drug scheduling, and enforcement of these laws.

Early notification of other stakeholders in parallel public health fields, such as drug treatment, harm reduction, emergency medicine, and social services, and public safety domains like border security, homeland security, supports enforcement and interdiction of novel substances enables all agencies to be better prepared and to respond more effectively, than when that information is received or shared later, or not at all. More comprehensive and informed forensic toxicology and seized drug testing will provide better, more timely information to other distribution channels reaching those groups, through organizations like the ASCLD, the NAME, the American College of Medical Toxicologists (ACMT), the National Drug Early Warning system (NDEWS), the New Jersey Drug Monitoring Initiative (NJDMI), and international groups like the European Monitoring Center for Drugs and Drug Addiction (EMCDDA), and the United Nations Office on Drugs and Crime (UNODC), and others.

Data science in forensic toxicology has been identified by the Toxicology Subcommittee of the OSAC as a research priority for the field. Data science—the consolidation and analysis large data sets, allows development of timely trend data, identifying the geographic origin of outbreaks of new drugs, emerging trends in drug combinations, co-occurrence of active drugs and precursor chemicals, and insights from retrospective data-mining, offer great insight into the origins, spread, and lifecycle of new substances, to name a few examples. This is an area that has not been exploited to date. Combining toxicology data with data from the autopsy, the scene investigation, and the decedents medical or drug use history, can give a better understanding of the significance of the drug findings in the context of lifestyle issues, drug tolerance, and ultimately lead to better informed determination of cause and manner of death. Combining medicolegal death investigation toxicology data with seized drug trends and drug use patterns in nonlethal intoxications in the emergency room, strengthen our understanding of drug threats even more.

There are other key areas where research is needed in forensic toxicology. This would include developing a better understanding of the extent of drug interactions at the receptor and metabolic level. The role of pharmacogenomic differences in metabolism resulting from polymorphisms in the enzymes responsible for drug metabolism need to be better understood, which will promote the adoption of pharmacogenomics considerations into drug interpretation.

More work should be done on the study of PMR. A lot of what we know about PMR is from work done in the 1980s and 1990s, when we didn't understand or measure how much of these site-dependent differences in drug concentration came from the uncertainty of measurement in the drug concentrations. Having better tools to characterize the limits of our analytical methods will give greater insight into what can be said about the potential for postmortem change in drug concentrations.

The OSAC toxicology subcommittee also identifies human factors considerations in toxicological analysis, and the significance of herbal and dietary supplements and plant-based toxins to toxicological analysis as areas ripe for more research.

11.4 Conclusion

Forensic toxicology was born in academic research laboratories at the turn of the twentieth century. It has strong roots in clinical laboratory science and is strongly supported by peer-reviewed literature and studies. It is an interdisciplinary endeavor with elements from chemistry, physics, biochemistry, anatomy and physiology, analytical chemistry, molecular biology, pharmacology, clinical toxicology, and statistics to name a few, and continues to be supported by research and productive collaborations with academic research centers. The profession is on a strong footing and has adapted well to face the challenges it will face.

We have many resources to support our growth and development, including a strong section in the AAFS, a warm, welcoming and professional resource in the SOFT, and international connections through TIAFT, among others.

The next 10 years will bring more change; stronger standards for accreditation, better and more powerful screening technologies, better interdisciplinary cooperation and communication, and more creative utilization of our big data sets. These changes will likely drive others, including more consolidation of resources, leading to better equipped, more appropriately staffed laboratories to address the workload demands and complexity of the testing.

Acknowledgments

I would like to acknowledge the many colleagues, peers, students, young scientists, researchers, and forensic toxicology enthusiasts who have shaped and continue to shape my growth in this exciting and rewarding field. My colleagues in the AAFS and other professional organizations, my fellow past presidents, and the young people I work with every day, whose energy, enthusiasm, hard work, and thirst for knowledge give me great hope for the future of forensic toxicology.

Index

AAFS Standards Board (ASB),
        69–70
adversarial system, 51, 53
age at death, 6–7
airplanes, 56
American Academy of Forensic
        Sciences (AAFS), 124–126
    General Section of, 61–62,
        71–72
    Jurisprudence Section of, 73–75
    QD Section task group on opinion
        terminology, 127–128
American Board of Forensic
        Document Examiners, Inc.
        (ABFDE), 126–127
American Board of Forensic
        Odontology, 95–96
American Board of Medicolegal
        Death Investigators
        (ABMDI), certification,
        66–68
American Board of Pathology
        (ABP), 108, 109
American Institute of Physics, 52
American National Standards
        (ANS), 69
American National Standards
        Institute (ANSI), 43, 69, 70
American Society of Questioned
        Document Examiners
        (ASQDE), 123–124
American Veterinary Medical
        Association (AVMA), 62
    policies of, 65
analytical toxicology, 157

ancestry, 9
anthropology, 1, 6
    age at death, 6–7
    ancestry, 9
    application, 3
    certification, 13
    date of death, 7–8
    detection and recovery, 3–4
    foul play, 11–12
    future progress, 13
    human status determination,
        4–5
    individual certification, 12–13
    living stature, 9–10
    positive individual identification,
        10–11
    sex estimation, 8–9
    taphonomy, 10
ASTM E444-09, 130
ASTM E30 Committee on Forensic
        Science, 128
ASTM Standard E2388-11, 130
automation, in forensic handwriting
        examination, 146–147
automobiles, 56

Barnes, Patrick MD, 52
big data, 36
biological weapons, 57
biometrics, 41
bitemark analysis, 93, 94, 105
black boxes, 56
body, stylized human, 57
Boise State University, 52, 53n
bones, 5, 12

The Future of Forensic Science, First Edition. Edited by Daniel A. Martell.
© 2019 John Wiley & Sons Ltd. Published 2019 by John Wiley & Sons Ltd.

Brain Research through Advancing
  Innovative
  Neurotechnologies® (BRAIN)
  initiative, 112
bullet lead analysis, 54
burden, legal, 50

cameras, 56
  identification, 40–41
carbon-14 dating, 7
cargo, 57
causal determinism, 116
CCTV cameras, 31
CEDAR-FOX, 146, 147
Center of Excellence for Document
  Analysis and Recognition
  (CEDAR), 138
certification, 126–127
  ABMDI, 66–68
  American Board of Medicolegal
    Death Investigators
    (ABMDI), 66–68
  FDE and Daubert standard, 135
  forensic anthropology, 12–13
  medicolegal death investigators,
    67
Chabot, Charles, 122
clinical evidence, 53
cloud computing, 43
cold fusion, 50
communication, electronic and
  otherwise, 56
communication surveillance, 57
Computer Aided Post Mortem
  Identification (CAPMI),
  99–100
computer-based forensic
  handwriting examination
  systems, 146–147
computerized axial tomography
  (CAT scan), 108
consciousness
  failure of physical sciences,
    115–116

hard problem of, 114–115
  theories of, 113–114
Consensus Bodies (CBs), 69
convictions, wrongful, 51
correlation *vs.* causation, 113
crime-lab forensic practice, 51
criminalistics
  definition, 19
  drug chemistry, 20
  financial burdens, 24–28
  fingerprint examination, 20
  firearm/toolmark examination,
    20
  forensic biology, 20
  forensic photography, 20
  quality issues, 23–24
  technological advances
    computer-driven systems,
      20–21
    databases and softwares, 20–21
    DNA technology, 21
    impression evidence, 21–22
    instrumentation, 22–23
    trace evidence, 20
criminal law and human mind,
  112–113

damaged (mobile) devices, 37–38
Daubert standard, 77, 133–141
Daubert v. Merrell Dow Pharma-
  ceuticals, Inc. (1993), 50
  Daubert test, 77
  history of, 75–77
  NAS report, 78–80
  questions raised, 77–78
death investigation, 157, 162, 169
deep learning, 39–40
defendants, 50
dental age assessment, 103–105
dental alloy/amalgam restorations,
  92
dental negligence (malpractice), 106
detection methods, 3–4

digital and multimedia sciences, 31,
32
challenges, 43–44
damaged (mobile) devices, 37–38
digital evidence, 35–37
disasters/large scale incidents, 42
drones, 41–42
geo satellites, 42
history of, 33–35
multimedia (*see* multimedia)
quality assurance, 43
sensors, 42
wearables and quantified self, 41
digital evidence, 35–37
digital X-ray imaging, 108
Disaster Mortuary Operational
Response Teams (DMORT),
99
disasters, 42
disguised writing, 142
disputes, civil, 56
DNA technology, 21, 51
double-aspect theory, 114
Doud, Donald, 125
drones, 41–42
drug chemistry, 20
drugs, 157–165, 169–171 *see also*
toxicology
due process, 70

education accreditation, 70–71
Edwards, Harry T., Hon., 51n
Electric Network Frequency (ENF),
40
engineering-science practitioners,
55
Engineering Sciences Section, 53
epiphenomenalism, 114
E30.02 Questioned Document
Subcommittee, 128–129
European Network of Forensic
Science Institutes (ENFSI),
37, 39
evidence-based legal medicine, 52

evidence-based medicine, 54
experiment, 54
expert testimony, 50
eye tracking study and FDEs,
144–145

Facial Identification Scientific
Working Group, 39
fingerprint examination, 20
firearm/toolmark examination,
20
FLASH-ID, 146, 147
forensic biology, 20
forensic document examination
(FDE), 119
civil cases, 121
and Daubert standard
certification, 135
error rate/reliability, 136–137
peer review and publication,
140–141
testing of basic principles,
137–140
eye tracking, 144–145
job description, 120
neuroscience, 142–144
operational standards, 130–133
forensic engineering sciences, 55n,
56, 57
Forensic Information System for
Handwriting (FISH), 138
forensic photography, 20
forensic psychiatry, 111
Forensic Science Education
Programs Accreditation
Commission (FEPAC), 70–71
Forensic Science Standards Board
(FSSB), 69, 82–83
Forensic Specialties Accreditation
Board (FSAB), 67
forensic subject-matter experts, 68
forensic veterinary science, 62–66
foul play, 11–12
free will, 116–117

Frye test, 76
Frye v. United States (1923), 76

gas chromatography–mass
    spectrometry (GCMS), 164
gatekeeper role, 51
General Electric Co. v. Joiner (1997),
    78
General Section, of AAFS, 61–62,
    71–72
genuine and disguised signatures,
    142
geo satellites, 42
Glick, Jill MD, 54
Gradwohl, Rutherford B.H., 73
Graphical Processing Units (GPUs),
    39

handwriting examination *see also*
    forensic document
    examination (FDE)
    automation, 146–147
    current research, 147–148
    discriminability of, 139
    of identical and fraternal twins,
        137
Harold A. Feder award, 75
Harvard Medical School, 52
higher-resolution satellite imaging
    systems, 42
high-resolution mass spectrometry
    (HRMS), 168
Hilton, Ordway, 124–126
Huber, P.W., 50
human mind and criminal law,
    112–113
human performance, 159, 163

idealism, 114
iFox, 147
impression evidence, 21–22
Inbau, Fred, 73–74
incarceration, 51
incompatibilism, 116

innocence, 51
interactionalism, 113
interdisciplinary knowledge
    sharing, 84
International Association of
    Forensic Sciences (IAFS), 126
International Law Enforcement
    Conference on Computer
    Evidence, 33
International Organization on
    Computer Evidence (IOCE),
    33
International Veterinary Forensic
    Sciences Association
    (IVFSA), 65, 66
internet, 57
interpretive toxicology, 157
ISIS, 57
isochrony principle, 143

judge, 50
junk law, 50, 51
junk science, 50
Jurisprudence Section, of AAFS,
    73–75

Kam, Moshe, 133, 136, 137
Kaye, Sidney, 73
Keep, Nathan Cooley, 91
King, Pamela A. W., 74
Kuhnian, 52
Kuhn, Thomas PhD, 52, 54, 54n
Kumho Tire Co. v. Carmichael (1999),
    78
Kurzweil, Raymond, 36

large scale incidents, 42
law and science interdisciplinary
    education, 86
Law Enforcement Assistance
    Administration (LEAA), 126
Leverhulme Research Centre for
    Forensic Science, 86

liquid chromatography/tandem
    mass spectroscopy
    (LCMSMS), 168
LODOX technology, 108

mail, 57
maintenance of certification (MOC)
    requirements, 109–110
mass spectrometry, 159, 164
materialism, 114
medicolegal death investigators,
    certification process for, 67
microprocessors, 56
Mind and Cosmos, 117
mobile devices
    damaged devices, 37–38
    sensors on, 42
multimedia, 38–39
    biometrics, 41
    camera identification, 40–41
    deep learning, 39–40

Nagel, Thomas, 117
naked passenger, 57
National Academy of Engineering,
    52
National Academy of Sciences
    (NAS) Report, 23–24, 51
    Daubert, 78–80
    for judicial and legal education,
        84–87
    NCFS, 80–82
    OSAC, 82–83
National Commission on Forensic
    Science (NCFS), 67, 74,
    80–82, 84, 85
National Institute for Standards and
    Testing (NIST), 166–167
National Institute of Justice (NIJ),
    166
National Institutes of Health, 52
National Research Council Report
    (2009), 51

National Technology Transfer and
    Advancement Act (NTTAA),
    70
neck injuries, 53
neural networks, 39
neuroscience and FDEs, 142–144
Newton's laws, 53, 54
NIST Forensics—Organization of
    Scientific Area Committees
    (OSAC), 96, 106
novel psychoactive substances
    (NPS), 163, 164
nutritionist, 64

occasionalism, 114
odontology/dentistry, 91, 92
    bitemark analysis, 93, 94, 105
    dental age assessment, 103–105
    dental misidentifications, 102
    dental negligence (malpractice),
        106
    digital record-keeping, 96–97
    personal abuse, 106
    practical issues, 95
    role in verifying victims identity,
        98
OdontoSearch®, 103
Ommaya, Ayub MD, 52
opioid crisis, 163
Organization of Scientific Area
    Committees (OSAC), 34, 43,
    82–84, 132, 133, 160, 167,
    171
    standards evolution, 68–69
    toxicology subcommittee, 167,
        171
Osborn, Albert S., 123–124

paradigm shift, 54, 55
parallelism, 114
pathological science, 50
pathology
    anatomic pathology, training
        requirement for, 108–109

pathology (*contd.*)
  computerized axial tomography
    (CAT scan), 108
  ideal/aspirational standards, 110
  LODOX technology, 108
  MOC requirements, 109–110
  overregulation by federal
    government, 110
  radiology technology, 107–108
  threats, 108–110
PCAST report (2016), 52
peer-reviewed publications, 50
perimortem, 12
perpetual motion, 50
Photo Response Nonuniformity
    (PRNU), 40
physical sciences, 115–116
plutonium, 57
poisons, 157–159 *see also* toxicology
Pollitt, Mark, 33
polywater, 50
postal services, international, 57
postmortem redistribution (PMR) of
    drugs, 160, 171
pre-established harmony, 114
privacy, data, 37
problem of free will, 116–117
product design, 55, 56
product-liability, 50, 56
Professional Science Masters (PSM)
    programs, 169
prosecutor, 50
public crime laboratory funding
  consolidation of laboratories,
    26–27
  cost recovery methods, 27–28
  grant funding, 25
  privatization, 28
  regionalization of services, 26
  staffing re-allocation, 25
Purtell, David J., 125

qualia, 115
quality assurance, 43, 160, 167

quantified self, 41
questioned document examination
    (QDE), origin of, 121–123 *see
    also* forensic document
    examination (FDE)

radiation, 57
radiocarbon dating, 104
radiology technology, 107–108
recovery efforts, 3–4
Reimann, Richard PhD, 53n
Resource Committees, FSSB, 83
retinal hemorrhages, 53
Richardson, Orville, 73
*The Role of the Courts in Improving
    Forensic Science* symposium,
    85
The Royal Society, 86

SBS theory *see* shaken baby
    syndrome (SBS) theory
scanning electron microscopy, 5
scientific approach, 54
Scientific Area Committees (SACs),
    68–69, 82, 83
scientific revolution, 52, 54
Scientific Working Group for
    Questioned Documents
    (SWGDOC), 129–132
Scientific Working group of Image
    Technology, 34
Scientific Working Groups (SWGs),
    68
scientist, 50
seaports, 57
security, 56
sensors, 42
sex estimation, 8–9
shaken baby syndrome (SBS)
    theory, 52–53
signature verification systems, 146
social media, 57
soft biometrics, 41
standardization, 33

ASTM International, 128–129
  opinion terminology, AAFS QD
    task group on, 127–128
  Scientific Working Group for
    Questioned Documents,
    129–130
standard reference material (SRM),
    164–165
standards evolution
  ASB, 69–70
  OSAC, 68–69
stature, 9–10
Structure of Scientific Revolutions, 55
subjective conscious experience,
    115
suitcase nuke, 57
surgical procedures, 56
SWG Medicolegal Death
    Investigations (SWGMDI), 68
Syndrome, The, 52

taphonomy, 10
Technical Working Group Digital
    Evidence (TWGDE), 33
Technical Working Group for
    Education and Training in
    Forensic Sciences (TWGED),
    71
Technical Working Group for
    Questioned Documents
    (TWGDOC), 129
terrorism, 56
terrorist attacks, 57
Thibault, Lawrence PhD, 52
time since death, 7–8

tombstone technology, 55
toxicology, 162
  analytical and interpretive, 157
  best practices recommendations,
    167
  data science, 170
  description, 157
  federal funds, 166
  laboratory resources, 166
  standards development, 166–167
trace evidence, 20
trauma, 12
triad, the, 53
trial by ordeal, 54

ugly American, 50n
Unified Victim Identification
    System–Case Management
    System (UVIS-CMS), 101
US Secret Service (USSS), 33
UVIS Dental Identification Module
    (UDIM), 101

validation, lack of, 51
validity, range of, 51
ventilation systems, 56
veterinary horse forensics, 63–64
voice-prints, 54

WANDA, 147
wearables, 41
Whitcomb, Carrie, 33, 34
WinID®, 100
Woodward, Louise, 52
workplace drug testing, 157, 162